A BRAIN SURGEON'S DISSECTION AND PRESCRIPTION

BITTER PILL

AMERICA AND HEALTHCARE IN AMERICA

OBAMACARE, ROMNEYCARE & MEDICARE (RYANCARE)

VIVEKANAND PALAVALI, M.D.

For more information about this title, please contact: www.bitterpilldoc.com

doc@surgeonscut.com

Book design by:

Blue Sun Press

Printed in the United States

BITTER PILL: America and Healthcare in America

Vivekanand Palavali, M.D.

1. Title 2. Author 3. Politics and Current Events/ Medical History I Law and Medicine/ Universal Healthcare

ISBN: 979-8-89669-038-2

Dedication

I am forever grateful to my father, whose compassion and kindness have been and will be an example to me, and my mother, whose patience and perseverance have been and will be inspirational.

I dedicate this book to my parents, as I respect them and cherish their love.

Acknowledgments

My journey to write this book actually started as a project to make the documentary film "*Bitter Pill: America and Healthcare in America.*" I met many men and women, young and old while making that film. They were generous with their time and willingness to talk to me about their experiences, fears, and hopes regarding healthcare in America. There are many I am grateful to, but I should especially thank some of them. Some of their names are changed for the sake of anonymity.

My gratitude should start with Whitney Gaines, whom I met as I was walking out of the Harvard University campus. She shared her heart-wrenching struggle with cancer and lack of adequate medical or monetary help. I am equally thankful to Iraq war veteran Sergeant William Kleinedler, who had to re-live his near-death experience from an IED[1] explosion in Iraq but didn't hesitate to talk about it.

I appreciate Dr. Arnold Relman for sparing some of his valuable time to talk about his experiences with the evolution of healthcare delivery in America and his insights into solving America's current healthcare problems.

I very much appreciate Dr. Margaret Flowers, whose commitment and activism to bring a single-payer system to America are commendable. She endured a chilly October morning in a tent at Freedom Plaza to talk with me after spending the entire previous day at the Annual Conference of Physicians for a National Health Program. I also met Dr. Alice Silverman and Dr. Ellen Oxfeld at the same conference. They enlightened me about their successful efforts to help bring about the first single-payer state in America. I admire and thank them. I must also thank Simon, Joe, Caren, Steve, Carol, and Geoff for taking the time in the middle of Occupy DC and peace marches to talk to me about their personal healthcare stories and their concerns about healthcare in America.

---

[1] Improvised explosive device

I thank Sherine and Omar for arranging to meet with Lona in Sweden. Lona and her husband adopted two orphan children from Africa. They invited me into their home and talked to me in detail about their personal journey into the adoption as well as the medical care they provided to those kids. Their hospitality and humanity will always be remembered, and I am very thankful.

Finally, I very much appreciate and thank Alexander P. Morgan for his editorial assistance as well as for editing the book in an expeditious manner.

Table Of Contents

Dedication ii

Acknowledgments iii

THE EMERGENCY 1

TWO AMERICAS 6

WORST BANG FOR THE BUCK 11

EVIL SOCIALIST SWEDEN 15

GATEWAY TO THE WEST 20

HIGHWAY TO HEALTHCARE HELL 23

SURGEON'S CUT 30

THE CANCER 35

HIPPOCRATES WHO? 40

AMBULANCE CHASERS 45

PLATINUM PILLS 49

LIFESTYLE AND LIFE 54

DEADLY DEVICES 58

MARGIN OVER MISSION 63

REAL DEATH PANELS 68

SENATORS FOR SALE 74

OBAMACARE 79

STOP SIGN AND THE INDIVIDUAL MANDATE 86

ROMNEYCARE 90

RYANCARE 93

BUDGET WARS 98

THE CURE 104

THE LITTLE ENGINE THAT COULD 112

LIFE, LIBERTY, AND THE PURSUIT OF HAPPINESS 118

"America's health care system is neither healthy, caring, nor a system."

–Walter Cronkite

Make no mistake. The cost of our health care is a threat to our economy. It's an escalating burden on our families and businesses. It is a ticking time bomb to the federal budget.

Barak Obama's Speech to the AMA

(American Medical Association) Chicago, Illinois, June 15, 2009

THE EMERGENCY

My beeper went off around 2:00 a.m. I was on call at a trauma center in Flint, Michigan, where I had been practicing neurosurgery for the past sixteen years. During those years, I was paged many times at all hours but never got used to being awakened from a deep sleep in the middle of the night—for who knows what emergency. I groaned with disappointment as I reached for the beeper. It had been a busy and long day of surgeries. But I was on call for neurosurgical emergencies, and that night, the page was about a head trauma.

A fifty-five-year-old man had tripped and fallen earlier in the evening. He had hit his head hard on a concrete floor and lost consciousness for a few minutes, but at the time, he refused to be taken to the emergency room. He complained of a headache before going to bed but told his wife he was going to sleep it off. When she woke up to go to the bathroom in the middle of the night, she found him unresponsive and gasping for air. She called 911, and the paramedics brought him to the emergency room of the hospital, where I was on call.

When I responded to the page, the neurosurgical physician assistant (PA) told me that the patient was deeply comatose and one of his pupils was blown, dilated, and not reacting to light, which meant that he was on the verge of death. A CAT[2] scan of his brain showed a large hematoma between the covering of the brain called the Dura and the brain itself, pushing the brain toward the opposite side of his skull. There was not much time to save his life. It truly was an emergency.

---

[2] Computed axial tomography

I told the PA to take the patient to the operating room and get him ready for surgery while I headed to the hospital. I performed a craniotomy, cut an opening in the skull, and removed the blood clot. After the surgery, I checked the pupil that had been dilated. It had become smaller and was now the same size as the other pupil. That was a good sign, but the patient's condition remained critical.

As I reviewed his information on the admission sheet to dictate the operative report, I noticed the words "private pay" in the box indicating insurance information. Those words were a polite way of saying he had no insurance. That might explain why he hesitated to come to the emergency room—but his hesitation had almost cost him his life.

Driving back home in the gloomy predawn dark, it was difficult to stay alert. I was exhausted, and a dense fog had rolled in, turning the familiar road into a blank, featureless landscape. Without the recognizable landmarks I usually relied on, finding my way ahead became a challenge. I couldn't stop thinking about the patient I had just operated on and all the Americans who, like him, lack health insurance. More than 47 million people in our country are uninsured, and when they face a medical emergency, their lives can become as desolate, dangerous, and uncertain as the road ahead of me that night.

*****

I completed my residency at the University of Chicago Hospitals in 1995 and began my practice as a neurosurgeon in Flint, Michigan. I worked at two hospitals with very different patient populations.

At one hospital, which was truly not-for-profit at the time, most of my patients were well-insured General Motors employees. After all, Flint was the "Vehicle City" and home to "Buick City" as well as the final assembly plant for General Motors trucks. These GM employees and retirees had comprehensive health insurance, including Blue Cross and Blue Shield (BCBS), which covered most of their medical expenses and provided fair compensation to doctors and hospitals.

The other hospital served a much larger population of indigent and poor patients. It had excellent pediatric and neonatal intensive care units and handled complicated pregnancies and deliveries. It was also a Level 1 trauma center, where I treated numerous cases of head trauma from automobile accidents, drunken bar brawls, and, of course, gunshot wounds—a grim reflection of Flint's reputation as one of the murder capitals of the country. This hospital received some financial assistance from the state because many of its patients were uninsured or on Medicaid. Medicaid, a state-funded insurance program for low-income individuals, didn't cover as much as premier private insurance policies.

I completed my residency at the University of Chicago Hospitals in 1995 and began practicing as a neurosurgeon in Flint, Michigan. I worked at two hospitals that catered to vastly different patient populations.

At one hospital, which was genuinely not-for-profit at the time, most of my patients were well-insured General Motors employees. After all, Flint was the "Vehicle City" and home to "Buick City" as well as the final assembly plant for General Motors trucks. These GM employees and retirees had comprehensive health insurance, including Blue Cross and Blue Shield (BCBS), which covered most of their medical expenses and ensured fair compensation for doctors and hospitals.

The other hospital served a significantly larger population of indigent and poor patients. It offered outstanding pediatric and neonatal intensive care units and handled complicated pregnancies and deliveries. It was also a Level 1 trauma center, where I treated numerous cases of head trauma resulting from automobile accidents, drunken bar brawls, and, of course, gunshot wounds—a grim reminder of Flint's reputation as one of the murder capitals of the country. This hospital received some financial support from the state because many of its patients were uninsured or on Medicaid. Medicaid, a state-funded insurance program for low-income individuals, didn't cover as much as the premier private insurance policies.

These days, Flint is a paradox to me as it strives to revive itself. Downtown has become artistic and vibrant, even boasting some good restaurants. The cultural center, with its Whiting Auditorium and institutes of music and art, has prospered. The annual summer "Back to Bricks" car show has grown increasingly crowded and enjoyable—if you can overlook the occasional gunshot wounds or the police clearing the streets due to a bomb threat. Yet, despite these recent changes suggesting a move toward prosperity, the Flint I see, from the perspective of affordable healthcare, remains in trouble. Many residents who were once comfortably employed and insured are now unemployed, poor, and without health coverage.

Interestingly, one of the hospitals in town didn't succumb to Flint's economic decline. In fact, the non-profit hospital has transformed into a highly profitable corporation. It introduced advanced but extremely expensive medical technologies to Flint and expanded its reach into a wider area of mid-Michigan. Unfortunately, the overall health of the community has deteriorated, and it has not benefited from the prosperity or expansion of this hospital corporation. Many residents can't afford even basic medical care, let alone these advanced technologies.

The rising costs of healthcare, the growing number of uninsured, and the resulting unequal quality of medical care between the rich and the poor are not problems unique to Flint. Nearby Motown, Detroit, has followed a similar trajectory. The Ford manufacturing center in Highland Park, just north of downtown Detroit, has also faced the fate of permanently locked gates. The police headquarters and fire station in Highland Park are dilapidated, standing as stark physical reminders of the broken economy and healthcare system.

This is not just a local issue; it is a crisis affecting every town and city in America. Escalating healthcare costs, spiraling out of control, are bankrupting communities—and the nation.

No wonder President Obama took notice of the critical condition of healthcare in America. He went to Chicago to seek the support of the American Medical Association, as well as the nation, to address the ailing American healthcare system.

Can Mr. Obama fix the broken system and rescue America's dying healthcare?

He recognized that this was an emergency, but I am not sure if he fully understood the magnitude and seriousness of the healthcare problem—or that there is an America within America.

*****

There are only three problems with healthcare in America: cost, quality, and access.

–John Goodman, Health Economist

TWO AMERICAS

I was stunned. I couldn't believe what I was seeing. I had just left the campus of Harvard University, and there on the street was a woman begging, holding a sign that read, "Cancer patient! Please help." She wore a headscarf to cover her hair loss, but unfortunately, it didn't fully do the job. Part of her bald head—typical of cancer patients undergoing chemotherapy—was visible. I couldn't miss the sadness etched on her face. It was unbelievable to see a cancer patient, an American no less, begging on the streets of Cambridge, Massachusetts, USA.

I had to stop and talk to her, which I did. Her name was Whitney Gaines. She was fifty years old and suffering from bladder cancer that had spread to her intestines. She wasn't sure if it had also reached her liver. As if that weren't enough, she also had Hepatitis C. Her voice choked, and her eyes welled with tears as she spoke.

She told me she had no family and no medical insurance. Thanks to Medicare and MassHealth, she was receiving some help and necessary treatments. However, she had to stop certain treatments because her body couldn't tolerate the chemotherapy. She didn't have enough money for food or even a train ticket to get to the hospital. As degrading as it was to beg on the streets, she said she had no choice. Without holding that sign and asking for help, she would have to eat garbage.

I never expected to hear such a story in America, the most powerful and one of the richest nations on earth.

As a neurosurgery resident training at the University of Chicago, I didn't have to worry about or know much about the patient's ability to pay for their healthcare. My focus was solely on taking care of the patients and honing my skills. However, when I started my own practice in Flint, I was quickly made aware of the financial realities of the medical world. I learned the harsh truth: millions of Americans cannot afford or access even basic healthcare.

According to the 2010 census, 50.7 million people in America were uninsured. In some states, more than 25% of the population lacked health insurance. These numbers are staggering. One out of every four residents in glitzy and glamorous California is uninsured. Similarly, one out of every four Texans—living in the oil-rich state famous for its Stetson-and-cowboy-boot-wearing tycoons—is also uninsured.

Within a few months of starting my practice, I couldn't ignore the stark reality that America operates with a two-tier healthcare system: one for the wealthy, with premier health insurance, and one for everyone else. A few uninsured patients receive help from charitable doctors and free clinics, like the Genesee Free Clinic in Flint. Others don't even have access to these resources. For them, the emergency room becomes both the first and the last resort for any and all medical problems. Tragically, many of these issues could be addressed earlier and more affordably by a family doctor or primary care provider—if these patients had the financial means or access to such care.

Unfortunately, many rural parts of America lack access to emergency rooms or free clinics. People in these areas rely on mobile free clinics provided by organizations like Remote Area Medical (RAM). RAM, founded by British doctor Stan Brock, was initially created to serve the sick poor in remote areas of third-world countries. Years ago, the majority of RAM's services were offered abroad, but today, over 65% of RAM's efforts are focused within the United States. This shift starkly illustrates how the state of healthcare in America has declined to a level comparable to that in some third-world countries, like India—a country I am quite familiar with.

*****

I was born in Madanapalle, a small town in southern India surrounded by rolling hills, small lakes, sugarcane fields, coconut trees, coconut-eating monkeys, and, of course, monkey gods. Did I mention cows and holy cows? My childhood was comfortable in this decent-sized town, but not too far away were many small villages where I witnessed what it truly means to be poor.

People in these villages worked extremely hard, performing back-breaking jobs just to earn enough for a day's worth of food. Poverty was evident in the eyes of the children, who walked barefoot for miles every day just to attend school. The landscape around these villages was picturesque, but basic facilities for hygiene and preventive health were nonexistent. Easily preventable diseases were widespread, and a lack of money made it difficult to treat even minor illnesses. Effective care for more serious conditions was generally unavailable in these rural areas.

Sadly, the situation hasn't improved much today. A few months ago, while visiting a small village near my hometown, I saw a man on the street with a tumor in his neck. I immediately suspected it was cancer of the thyroid gland. I spoke with him, and he told me he had tried to seek help at a teaching hospital seventy miles away—the same hospital where I went to medical school and completed my clinical training.

He was admitted and waited several days for a specialist to see him, but the doctor never came from the nearby city. It was too expensive and difficult for his family to stay at the hospital far from home for more than a few days, so he had no choice but to return home without receiving the care he needed. When I think about the slow and painful death he may face, I feel deeply sorry for him.

The hospital where I completed my clinical training is a government hospital. Its funding comes from the state government and the estate of the second richest god in the world, whose temple sits atop the hill next to the hospital. While the care provided is free, it primarily addresses common illnesses. If a wheelchair isn't available, your family members become your crutches. They are also your transporters if you have an accident, as there are not enough ambulances.

If you are poor but fortunate enough to be admitted, you might receive necessary treatment for less complex ailments. However, if you suffer from a major illness, you may be forced to accept that your life is at risk. Many other government-run hospitals face similar inadequacies. On the other hand, if you are wealthy, you can travel to cities with corporate hospitals that rival those in America. These facilities offer state-of-the-art medical care, including knee replacements with imported artificial joints, performed by doctors trained in the United States or Europe.

It's as if there are two Indias when it comes to healthcare: one for the rich, who receive clean, private rooms and modern medicine, and another for the poor, who endure dirty common wards that may not even provide basic care. The poor must make do, like the man I saw during my last visit a few months ago, begging outside the hospital where I trained. He had lost a finger to a minor infection and his wife to an obstetric complication—both likely preventable. Instead, he now begs on the streets.

As heartbreaking as it is, medical beggars are not an uncommon sight in India. But what shocked me was seeing Whitney begging on the streets of Cambridge, Massachusetts. Lack of healthcare or support for the suffering poor is expected in a developing country like India, which could benefit from organizations like Remote Area Medical (RAM). However, it is hard to fathom that America, the premier first-world country, also needs RAM's services—just like many third-world nations.

RAM, true to its name, was originally created to serve people in need in remote rural areas. However, it has come to recognize the harsh reality that inadequate access to healthcare in America is not limited to rural areas. Due to uncontrollable and spiraling medical costs, many hospitals in urban areas have been forced to close their doors permanently.

I recall seeing a hospital in East St. Louis with its main entrance boarded up, now standing as a sad relic of an institution that once healed the sick and brought new life into the world. While such a fate may not be surprising for a hospital in a poor city like East St. Louis, the closure of a prominent and well-loved facility like St. Vincent's Hospital in Queens, New York, is startling. This is why RAM now operates not only in rural areas of poor states like Tennessee but also in urban centers like Los Angeles, California.

People line up for hours, sometimes enduring cold nights, to receive free medical care. They might be seeking a routine physical, an eye exam for glasses, or desperately needed dental work. Others come for help with chronic conditions like diabetes or hypertension. These easily treatable problems can become life-threatening without care, leading to devastating strokes or kidney failure.

What astonishes me is that many RAM patients are insured but not adequately insured. Seeing pictures of desperate Americans waiting in long lines for basic medical care reminds me that, just like in India, there are two Americas when it comes to accessing and affording healthcare.

The number of free clinics—and the number of Americans relying on them—has steadily increased across this great first-world nation. Yet, many people are still turned away by these clinics, which cannot handle the overwhelming healthcare needs of the uninsured and underinsured. The Genesee Free Clinic in Flint, for instance, has witnessed this growing demand for free healthcare.

It's not that America doesn't spend money on healthcare. It spends an extraordinary amount—nearly $3 trillion. With that level of expenditure, it's reasonable to expect that all Americans would have access to basic healthcare.

This raises the million-dollar—or rather, trillion-dollar—question: America is footing an enormous healthcare bill, so why isn't it getting the best possible deal for its money?

*****

Let's get this straight. America is the only industrialized nation in the world that does not guarantee healthcare to all of its citizens.

–Bernie Sanders, Independent Senator from Vermont

WORST BANG FOR THE BUCK

$7.7 Trillion!

That is the staggering amount projected to be the cost of healthcare in America in 2022. It exceeds the combined GDPs of Russia, Canada, India, Spain, and Australia.

In 1980, the cost of healthcare in America was $256 billion. By 2010, it had skyrocketed to $2.6 trillion, amounting to 17.1% of GDP in 2011. Current projections only show this number increasing. Yet, despite the vast sums spent on healthcare, basic healthcare is not provided to all Americans, nor are Americans healthier than the citizens of other developed nations.

In 2000, the World Health Organization conducted a survey of its 191 member countries, evaluating:

1. How a nation improves the health of its citizens.
2. Reduces health disparities.
3. Protects households from impoverishment due to medical expenses.
4. Provides responsive services that respect the dignity of patients.

France ranked first in the survey, while America ranked 30th. Not only do all other industrialized nations rank ahead of America in terms of the health of their citizens, but they also achieve better outcomes at half the national medical expenditure.

At a cost of $8,000 per person, American healthcare is two and a half times more expensive than the average for OECD (Organization for Economic Co-operation and Development) countries, which include the U.S., France, Finland, Germany, Japan, Sweden, Canada, the UK, Denmark, and 25 other nations. Japan, which spends just $2,000 per capita, boasts the best life expectancy among OECD countries.

Shockingly, a baby born in America has better chances of survival in 38 other nations; the U.S. ranks 39th in the world for infant mortality. Adults fare no better. America ranks 43rd in adult female mortality, 42nd in adult male mortality, and 36th in life expectancy.

It is alarming that the wealthiest nation on earth lags so far behind other developed countries when it comes to the health and well-being of its people.

The other sad truth, as Senator Sanders lamented, is that despite spending more on healthcare than the entire GDPs of several major countries, America has failed to provide basic healthcare for all its citizens. This first-world democracy, "of the people, by the people, and for the people," has fallen short when it comes to ensuring decent healthcare access for *all* the people.

Meanwhile, many Western European industrialized nations have provided universal healthcare to their citizens for decades: England since 1948, Japan since 1938, Germany since 1941, Sweden since 1955, and France since 1974. Surveys and studies show that citizens in these countries are generally satisfied and happy with their healthcare systems. In stark contrast, America seems unable to get the best value for the extraordinary amount it spends on healthcare.

How do so many countries provide universal healthcare at a reasonable cost? Can America learn from them? The answer to that seems to be a resounding *No!* Many Americans resist the idea of following the lead of other nations, particularly Western European countries that are perceived as being too socialist. Americans take pride in their individualism and are often skeptical of government involvement in their lives.

For many, the perception is that European governments are too large, tax their citizens excessively, and limit personal freedom, choice, and alternatives. But where do Americans get this impression? What shapes the narrative that leaves them so opposed to adopting lessons from systems that seem to work better elsewhere?

I think the answer to that question becomes obvious to anyone who listens to the politicians and political pundits dominating the airwaves and broadcast TV. As for the political pundits, I am certain that some of them are paid—directly or indirectly—to say what they say. But are these "expert" pundits truly experts, or are they simply spouting unfounded opinions? I doubt many of them have ever personally spoken to citizens in other countries about their healthcare systems. Who knows what hidden agendas they may have? I wouldn't be surprised if their rhetoric is primarily aimed at advancing their own self-interests.

As for the politicians, particularly Republicans, they often argue that government is inherently bad and that private citizens should handle things without government regulation or oversight. They equate government expansion—even when it is clearly necessary—with Europeanization, claiming it would result in limited choices, diminished freedoms, and a lack of alternatives.

But are these politicians genuinely expressing the truth as they see it, or are they demonizing socialized healthcare systems in industrialized Western European countries for their own political advantage in America?

One thing is clear: we can't take everything politicians say at face value or assume their words are always in the best interest of the citizens. They are, after all, politicians! Many insist that Americans have the best healthcare system in the world. Either they are lying, or they have no clue about the reality of healthcare in this country.

I have been taking care of patients in America for twenty-two years, including six years of training. From my experience, it doesn't feel like these anti-universal-healthcare politicians are talking about the same people I see in my office every day—people who are uninsured, underinsured, or unable to afford the medications and medical devices they need for a healthy and happy life.

These politicians argue that in socialist countries like Sweden, people have to endure long waits for medical care, even for treatments addressing painful conditions. They label these countries as "evil." But I wonder—have many of our politicians ever been to Sweden or even spoken to a Swede? Figuratively speaking, it feels like visually impaired politicians and pundits are leading the blind American public when it comes to discussions about healthcare in Western European nations.

Instead of relying on the opinions of politicians and pundits, I wanted to find out for myself what the citizens of these "evil" socialized European countries truly thought and felt about their healthcare systems. I decided I needed to speak directly with Swedish people and doctors. Perhaps then, I could determine whether a less wealthy Scandinavian socialist country like Sweden actually meets the healthcare needs of all its citizens.

So, I went to Sweden.

*****

It is good. We still have a lot of freedoms and choices. It is good to have the security.

–A happy Swedish citizen

EVIL SOCIALIST SWEDEN

Lona is a gentle soul. She is married to Mike, and they have a beautiful daughter together. However, Lona always dreamed of adopting children. Her father was born in Morocco but later migrated to Sweden, where Lona was born. A few years ago, she realized her wish by adopting two boys, Kaleb and Ashraf, from an orphanage in Addis Ababa, Ethiopia. It was as if her ancestral land of Africa had called her to extend a helping hand to its less fortunate children.

The first time I saw Kaleb in Lona's home in Stockholm, he was dancing to a Britney Spears song in the living room. Every time he turned his head to the right, I caught a glimpse of an oval-shaped, dark gray, shiny object implanted through his skull just behind his left ear—a cochlear implant. Without it, he wouldn't have been dancing.

Kaleb was born deaf, something Lona and her husband were aware of before adopting him and bringing him to Sweden from Ethiopia. In Sweden, he was fitted with a hearing aid for his right ear and underwent surgery to receive the cochlear implant in his left ear. According to Lona, the implant allowed Kaleb to hear better, learn to speak, and even enjoy music. It brought joy and rhythm into his life, enabling him to dance.

A few years later, they adopted their second son, Ashraf, who had a serious illness—one that likely would have been fatal if he had remained in Ethiopia. Today, Ashraf is a healthy, lively, and lovable child.

I was deeply inspired by the compassion, love, and courage of Lona and her husband. They made an extraordinary difference in the lives of two children who were born into unfortunate circumstances but given a second chance by two kind and selfless people.

Because of the medical challenges her boys were born with, Lona had to immerse herself in the Swedish healthcare system. She was gracious enough to share her experiences with me.

*****

When I landed in Stockholm, I was greeted at the airport—not by the actual King and Queen of Sweden, but by pictures of the royal family, along with images of my childhood favorites, Bjorn Borg and ABBA. The city itself is not very large, but it is clean, friendly, and safe. In the three days I spent there, I didn't see a single police car. However, I did come across a striking metal statue of a revolver with its barrel tied into a knot, located in the heart of a popular shopping district. I suppose the Swedes don't have much of an affinity for guns—perhaps one reason the city isn't violent.

Stockholm also struck me as a remarkably tolerant city. In the middle of a bustling shopping area, I saw a large photograph in a store window depicting two men kissing. I had never seen such an image displayed publicly in any American city.

On the day I was scheduled to meet Lona, she picked me up at my hotel and drove me to her home. After dinner, we sat down and talked. Lona shared the medical challenges her sons faced and how the Swedish government had taken care of all the expenses for Kaleb's deafness, including the surgery for his cochlear implant and the life-saving medications Ashraf needed.

But that wasn't all. Kaleb was enrolled in a special school for deaf children, and all his educational needs were fully funded by the government. Additionally, the government compensated Lona for the extra time she had to spend helping Kaleb with his learning due to his hearing disability.

I was amazed. I couldn't help but wonder how the Swedish government could afford to cover all these costs. My first thought was that Mike and Lona must be paying exorbitantly high taxes. So, I asked Mike how much they paid.

He explained that the average Swedish citizen pays about 30% in taxes, and the wealthy pay closer to 50%.

Really? I pay 50% of my income in taxes in America and still have to shell out significant additional money for medical insurance.

Here's another surprise: that 30% tax paid by Lona and Mike—both graphic designers—will also cover their kids' college tuition, including university education. Meanwhile, despite paying half my income in taxes in America, I don't receive that benefit. I still have to set aside money in a college fund for my boys.

I wondered if taxpayer-funded healthcare and education in Sweden came with limitations—perhaps a lack of choice in doctors or too many restrictions. Contrary to the common misconceptions in America, fueled by misinformation about government-run healthcare systems like Sweden's, Lona and Mike assured me that they have the freedom to choose their doctors.

Lona also shared a poignant observation: she had spoken to some American mothers with deaf children who couldn't afford cochlear implants. She was heartbroken to learn that in America, poor or middle-class deaf children often have no choice when it comes to receiving an implant—money decides for them. If you're deaf and lack the financial means in America, you may never hear music in your life.

It's true that Swedes might have to wait a little longer than they'd like for some elective surgeries. However, given the overall benefits of their healthcare system, they don't seem to mind. Lona shared the story of a man who waited several months for hip replacement surgery. That man happened to be the prime minister of Sweden, and he waited just like every other citizen. Now, that is what I call true democracy, equality, and justice.

I also asked about waiting lists for organ transplants. Lona explained that children are given priority over adults. I find it admirable to prioritize giving children a chance to live and experience life. Adults understand that they've already had more lives than those children, and such "rationing" seems reasonable.

It made me wonder: in America, is healthcare "rationed" not by need or fairness but by money and power?

Whether one labels Swedish society as "socialist" or not, its healthcare and social systems undeniably seem compassionate and caring. In Sweden, if someone becomes homeless—often due to mental illness or drug addiction—they are still eligible for and receive the same healthcare benefits as the country's prime minister. Remarkably, even outpatient psychiatric needs for the homeless are covered by the government. In contrast, many private insurance companies in America—highly profitable enterprises—do not cover psychiatric treatments at all.

I thanked Lona and Mike for their warm hospitality and the wealth of information they shared. Mike kindly offered to drop me back at my hotel. On the way, he took me to visit the largest public hospital in Stockholm, the prestigious Karolinska Institute. As we passed the emergency room of the Lindgren Pediatric Hospital, located next to Karolinska, Mike shared something astonishing. He explained that if he had to take his daughter to the emergency room in the middle of the night, it would cost him maybe $20. However, if he took her to a doctor's office the next day, the visit wouldn't cost him a single cent. It's simply unbelievable what the Swedes receive in exchange for the 30% taxes they pay.

During the car ride, I brought up the philosophical debate in America about individual freedom versus the role of government. I asked Mike what he thought about the differences between capitalist America and socialist Sweden. His response was simple: he was happy with their system. He said it felt good to have the security of quality healthcare, higher education, and safe streets—all provided by their socialist structure.

Now, can someone please explain to me why some of our politicians label Sweden an "evil socialist country"? Do they not see the injustice in American society, where access to quality healthcare or higher education at a prestigious university is reserved only for the wealthy?

How did America—the pioneer of democracy, the beacon of hope for people around the world, the most powerful and wealthiest nation on Earth, the country that put the first man on the moon—end up denying millions of its own citizens a healthy, prosperous, productive, and happy life?

This is not the America I remember from my youth, growing up in India.

*****

The test of our progress is not whether we add more to the abundance of those who have much; it is whether we provide enough for those who have too little.

–Franklin Delano Roosevelt

GATEWAY TO THE WEST

My first memory of America comes from when I was nine years old. I distinctly remember, even after so many years, the image that remains imprinted deep in my mind. It is the picture of Neil Armstrong standing on the moon, with the endless darkness of space in the background and the reflection of an American flag on the glass visor of his space helmet. Another image I will never forget is the imprint of a human step on the moon dust that was *"one small step for a man, a giant leap for mankind."*

I treasured those pictures. I cut them from magazines and placed them in my scrapbook of the first man on the moon. Every time I looked at them, they reminded me of the innovation, adventure, incredible achievement, and greatness of America.

Over the next few years, my impression of the riches of America was shaped by the Hollywood movies I watched in my hometown almost every Sunday morning. The tall, shiny skyscrapers in cities like New York and Chicago and the roads filled bumper to bumper with cars made me imagine how wealthy America was. I had already heard rumors that there was no poverty in America and that everyone was rich and owned one or more cars. From watching the movies, I assumed all of those rumors were true.

I came to St. Louis in 1986. I remember going to the banks of the Mississippi and Missouri rivers near downtown and seeing, for the first time, the gigantic silver-metal arch reflecting the sun as if lighting the way to the west. Just as St. Louis was the gateway to the West for early explorers from the East in America, it became the gateway to the Western world for me, coming from the Eastern world.

My initial impression was that America was a great country! I was amazed by the big, beautiful homes in clean subdivisions, the rich and luxurious shopping malls, the opulence all around, and, of course, cars everywhere. There were so many cars that the highways were congested, and at times, the traffic came to a standstill. In India, we had a different reason for coming to a complete stop on the roads: the natural, moving speed breakers—buffalos, cows, and goats. They didn't brake for you! You had to brake for them. It didn't matter how much you honked your horn; they didn't give a damn. You just had to stop and let them have the right of way.

What amazed me the most were the incredible highways in America and the fact that you could travel from one end of the country to the other on the interconnected interstate highways without stopping. Needless to say, I felt the grass sure was greener in America, that every American was rich, and that there was no poverty.

That's what I thought until one day when I took a wrong exit and ended up in East St. Louis. That's when I had my first glimpses of the poor, dirty, and ugly side of America. I was exposed to a part of America I never imagined existed when I was a boy growing up in India.

Twenty-five years later, on a foggy, dreary morning in 2011, I returned to East St. Louis. It felt like a ghost town and looked worse than I remembered. The roads were deserted, with no cars or pedestrians. Some stores were permanently boarded up, while others were gated for security. I saw abandoned gas stations and fish markets, a man living under a bridge, and a burned-out church whose facade had collapsed to the ground. Now, it was nothing more than a pile of bricks, with weeds growing everywhere. Even the house of God had not escaped the wrath of poverty.

I also came across a dilapidated, abandoned brick hospital building. A wall once adorned with large metallic letters spelling the hospital's name now bore only their shadows; the letters were long gone. Standing there, I couldn't help but feel the irony in that dead hospital. To me, it symbolized the state of healthcare in America today—critical, deteriorating, and dying.

What historical path did this great nation take to end up in its current unfortunate state?

*****

Of all forms of inequality, injustice in healthcare is the most shocking and inhumane.

—Martin Luther King

HIGHWAY TO HEALTHCARE HELL

Early in the twentieth century, patients in the United States received healthcare primarily from doctors in their clinics. People rarely went to hospitals. Doctors also made house calls, visiting the homes of the sick in an attempt to heal them as they lay in their own beds. Patients with money paid what the doctor charged, while those who were poor paid what they could. Doctors didn't mind; they were genuinely interested in healing the sick. Many physicians believed that answering the call to help the ill—rich or poor—was the very reason they had become doctors in the first place.

The practice of medicine in the late nineteenth and early twentieth centuries was relatively simple. It was more of an art than a science, as there were no effective remedies for many ailments. The agents responsible for diseases were just beginning to be understood. Louis Pasteur's research supported the theory that germs caused some diseases. Robert Koch founded modern microbiology by identifying the bacterial agents of tuberculosis, cholera, anthrax, and others. Joseph Lister studied the cause of sepsis and developed aseptic techniques, which became routine in-home treatment as well as in hospitals.

As medicine developed into more of a science, people began to benefit from having their illnesses treated in hospitals. Hospitals grew in popularity and became busier but remained nonprofit institutions. Hospital administrators performed their roles as managers, not as CEOs. At the time, there was no health insurance, and employers were not responsible for the healthcare costs of their employees. However, hospitals eventually began facing financial difficulties because many patients could not afford to pay for their care.

In 1929, Justin Ford Kimball, vice president of Baylor University's health facilities, introduced the concept of healthy people paying the hospital in advance for a promise of medical care (hospital expenses) if and when they got sick. Thus, the first prepaid health insurance to cover hospital expenses was born at Baylor University in Dallas, Texas. This plan guaranteed twenty-one days of hospital care for a $6 premium per year. Initially, it was offered to schoolteachers, later extended to other employee groups, and eventually made available to anyone interested and able to pay.

Anticipating competition among individual hospitals for enrollees, the hospital association grouped many such plans together under the Blue Cross system. This allowed patients who purchased insurance to choose their hospitals and doctors. Within a decade, the number of enrollees surged from 1,300 to 3,000,000, leading to the formation of a national American Hospital Association. In 1972, the Blue Cross Association separated from the American Hospital Association.

The first Blue Shield Plan was established in 1939 in California to cover physicians' fees. By 1948, nine such plans merged to form the Associated Medical Care Plan, later renamed the National Association of Blue Shield Plans. In 1982, Blue Shield merged with Blue Cross to create the Blue Cross and Blue Shield Association (BCBSA).

Until 1986, the Blue Cross system operated as a nonprofit and was tax-exempt. However, its success spurred the creation of many for-profit commercial health plans. In 1994, BCBSA changed its rules to allow member plans to become for-profit corporations. Since then, some BCBS member insurance plans have grown into massive profit-oriented corporations. These commercial insurance plans often aim to generate revenue from people's medical needs, sometimes by limiting benefits when enrollees fall ill.

WellPoint, the largest BCBS member plan, operates in 14 states and is a for-profit, publicly traded company. Meanwhile, BCBS of Michigan, which covers the medical needs of two out of every three

Michiganders in some form, is technically nonprofit. However, many Americans cannot afford the premiums for most insurance plans, whether commercial or nonprofit.

Over a century ago, some compassionate citizens in the United States were deeply concerned about the inability of many people to pay for medical care. These individuals sought to create a national health insurance system. Initially, they succeeded in convincing states to cover the costs of work-related injuries through workers's compensation. Encouraged by this progress, they championed the cause of a universal national health insurance system.

Unfortunately, this humane and progressive idea was widely perceived as socialist by many Americans, who were highly individualistic, skeptical of government, and staunch advocates of capitalism. Among the vocal opponents of nationalized health insurance was the American Medical Association (AMA). Its member physicians feared that such a system would limit their autonomy, reduce their income, and interfere with the doctor-patient relationship. While a minority of doctors supported the idea, their voices were drowned out by the majority.

Woodrow Wilson also opposed universal health insurance, and the cause lacked national political champions until Franklin Delano Roosevelt. In the 1930s, FDR wanted to include health insurance coverage for the elderly as part of Social Security. However, doctors' associations once again opposed the proposal, fearing government regulation of their services and incomes. As a result, the Social Security Act was passed without provisions for health insurance for the elderly and disabled.

Later, in 1949, the AMA played a pivotal role in defeating the proposed Murray-Wagner-Dingell bill, which would have provided nationalized health insurance for all Americans. To oppose this legislation, the AMA even charged its members $25 each to fund lobbying efforts. As a result, the frail elderly and disabled had to wait several more decades for government-provided medical insurance. It wasn't until 1965 that Medicare finally came into being.

In the early decades of the twentieth century, employer-provided health benefits were rare, and there were few private commercial medical enterprises offering diagnostic or ancillary medical services such as physical therapy or home health services. That was the state of healthcare in America before World War II.

Two significant events were primarily responsible for transforming the traditional way of delivering healthcare—where employer-provided health insurance was rare—into the current system, where many Americans receive employer-provided health benefits, and numerous for-profit ancillary medical enterprises, such as diagnostic radiology centers and laboratories, have emerged.

The first major event began with the bombing of Pearl Harbor and America's involvement in World War II. In response to the escalating demand for labor, Congress, at the urging of FDR, passed a law preventing wage increases. To attract workers in a competitive labor market, employers began offering health coverage as an incentive since they were prohibited from offering higher wages. Around the same time, advancements in diagnostic technology and the development of new drugs made medical care more expansive—and also more expensive. Those with employer-provided health insurance, however, had no trouble accessing as much healthcare as they needed.

The second—and most impactful—change that led to rising healthcare costs was the introduction of Medicare. President Truman had tried but failed to pass legislation for a national health insurance program. Lyndon Johnson, however, succeeded in passing the Medicare Act. Its purpose was to ensure the elderly and disabled could have their medical needs met. While this was an honorable and humane idea, enterprising capitalists quickly recognized the financial opportunity. Billions of dollars were about to flow into healthcare, creating a lucrative market.

This led to the establishment of the first "for-profit" private hospitals. Soon after, laboratories, diagnostic centers, physical therapy practices, and nursing homes—also for-profit enterprises—emerged. Thus, the "medical-industrial complex" was born.

Dr. Arnold S. Reiman, former chief editor of the prestigious *New England Journal of Medicine* and a professor of medicine and public health at Harvard Medical School, sounded the alarm in his 1980 article, *"The New Medical-Industrial Complex."* He compared this emerging system to the "military-industrial complex" that President Eisenhower warned about in his 1961 farewell address.

Dr. Reiman wrote:

"*The most important healthcare development of the day is the recent, relatively unheralded rise of a huge new industry that supplies healthcare services for profit. Proprietary hospitals and nursing homes, diagnostic laboratories, home-care and emergency-room services, hemodialysis, and a wide variety of other services produced a gross income to this industry last year of about $35 billion to $40 billion. This new 'medical-industrial complex' may be more efficient than its nonprofit competition, but it creates the problems of overuse and fragmentation of services, overemphasis on technology, and 'cream-skimming,' and it may also exercise undue influence on national health policy. In this medical market, physicians must act as discerning purchasing agents for their patients and therefore should have no conflicting financial interests. Closer attention from the public and the profession, and careful study, are necessary to ensure that the 'medical-industrial complex' puts the interest of the public before those of its stockholders.*"

Despite warnings from figures like Dr. Reiman, the use of expensive medical technologies to diagnose and advanced interventions to treat illnesses—including surgeries, medical devices, prosthetics, pharmaceuticals, physical therapy, nursing, and home healthcare services—has grown exponentially since Medicare's introduction.

The same belief that market forces will self-regulate, which underpins the evolution of all industries in America's capitalistic economy, has been applied to healthcare. Unfortunately, much like in other private, for-profit industries, the implicit goal of most medical enterprises has become maximizing profit while delivering care.

The result is *more* care—not necessarily the *most effective* care—partly because the more care provided, the more the provider gets paid, whether it's a primary doctor, surgeon, ambulatory surgical center, hospital, or any other ancillary medical service. This system is known as "fee-for-service."

As many healthcare providers are compensated based on the quantity of care rather than the quality, it is unsurprising to see diagnostic and therapeutic interventional procedures duplicated. Often, expensive interventions with no proven efficacy are approved and utilized. It is also common to see costly technology being employed, even when a less expensive but equally effective alternative is available.

The unrestricted use of medical care, combined with the proliferation of expensive pharmaceuticals and state-of-the-art technical innovations—some inadequately tested for their efficacy—has led to an inevitable escalation in medical costs over the past few decades. By 2011, healthcare expenditures had skyrocketed to $2.6 billion, as mentioned earlier.

Adding to the crisis is a lack of preventive services and a prevalence of unhealthy lifestyles, which has contributed to an uncontrolled epidemic of obesity. This has only exacerbated the problems created by the medical-industrial complex, further straining the system. The American healthcare delivery system is now buckling under its own weight.

At one point, private insurance HMOs attempted to manage rising medical costs through managed care. However, these efforts faced significant backlash from the American public, which strongly opposed the restrictions on "choice" imposed by HMO companies.

In response to uncontrolled medical costs, insurance companies have not only resorted to raising premiums but also frequently restrict or deny benefits to patients who believe those benefits are covered. Many others have been denied insurance or dropped from their existing coverage when they needed it most, often under the pretense of "pre-existing conditions." It is no surprise, then, that serious conflict has arisen between patients and profit-driven commercial health insurance companies.

The medical-industrial complex has become increasingly fragmented and highly commercialized, driven by an unchecked pursuit of profits. Patients with financial resources can afford healthcare, while those without must rely on charity, free clinics, or emergency room visits—or, worse, simply go without care.

How is it that an intelligent, compassionate, resilient, and innovative democracy—the same one that sent Voyager beyond the boundaries of the solar system—cannot stop healthcare delivery from sliding down the slippery slope into healthcare hell?

As a surgeon with an inquisitive mind and a drive to comprehensively understand complex issues, I felt compelled to dissect and diagnose the root cause of this problem. Why have physicians, politicians, leading citizens, and lawmakers been unable to prevent the regrettable deterioration of healthcare in America?

*****

What the mind doesn't know, the eye can't see.

–Anonymous

SURGEON'S CUT

First, there was some mid-back pain. She took over-the-counter pain medication, assuming it would go away. It didn't. Gradually, the pain worsened, and a few days later, she noticed her legs were becoming weaker. She felt slightly feverish, and her leg weakness progressed. She had to use a walker. Soon after, she developed numbness from the waist down. Then, she lost control of her bladder and couldn't stop herself from wetting.

She was brought to the hospital, and I was called for an urgent consultation. When I saw her, she was lying on her back, staying as still as possible because any movement caused agonizing back pain. She could barely move her legs and had severe tenderness when I pressed on the mid part of her spine. From these symptoms, I immediately suspected an infection of the spine with spinal cord compression—a neurological emergency.

A stat MRI confirmed the diagnosis: *discitis,* an infection of the cartilaginous disc between two vertebrae, along with *osteomyelitis,* an infection of the vertebrae. The infection had softened the bone, which collapsed and pushed part of the vertebra backward, compressing the spinal cord. This inescapable compression of her spinal cord was causing the rapid loss of function in her body below that level.

What would be the appropriate treatment in a case like this to prevent further deterioration and help the patient regain as much function as possible?

One can give Tylenol for fever, manage pain with powerful painkillers, and attempt to improve strength with good physical therapy, but none of that will matter unless the spinal cord compression is relieved and the deep-seated infection is eradicated. Simply treating the symptoms is futile; the patient will continue to deteriorate and could even die despite the high cost of managing her superficial symptoms. Surgery is required to remove the infected disc and vertebrae, eradicate the infection, decompress the spinal cord, and reconstruct the spine using strong metallic instrumentation. A condition this complicated and serious demands rapid and aggressive intervention if there is to be any hope of recovery.

Metaphorically speaking, healthcare in America is in a similarly critical condition. To effectively treat our failing healthcare system, we must diagnose the deep-seated "infection" that is eating away at it. The deeper I delve to uncover the root cause of this dysfunction and the intervention necessary to address it, the more apparent it becomes that the industry of healing the sick in America is incredibly complicated.

It is not just about doctors and nurses doing their jobs. Technology, innovation, enterprise, business, and politics—including foreign policy—are all interconnected in a complex, intricate web. This reminds me of a saying I once heard in India about water lilies: *"When you pull a vine, the entire swamp moves."*

Much of what is wrong with healthcare in America is happening beneath the surface, invisible to the unsuspecting patient. Some of the things occurring behind the scenes are not pleasant. Even some doctors are unaware of this complexity or are unwilling to acknowledge the darker side of healthcare delivery. No wonder the public, largely unaware of the "business" behind medicine, is confused about why healthcare in America is so dysfunctional!

There is one pervasive, crucial element infesting the medical industry that is primarily responsible for this dysfunction. To understand this infestation, it is helpful to trace the rise and fall of some of America's major industries and examine the recent trajectory of the American economy.

When I was training to be a neurosurgeon, I didn't know much about the unhealthy side of healthcare in America. My focus was entirely on mastering my specialty. However, once I began practicing in Michigan, I started to encounter aspects of the medical profession that troubled me deeply. Over the years, I repeatedly came across incidents and business practices that made me pause and reflect on the unfortunate reality of certain facets of the American healthcare system.

These experiences, along with my work as a practicing neurosurgeon, helped me connect the dots and understand the larger interconnected picture of medicine, business, politics, and the national economy. Moreover, as I witnessed the overall decline of the American economy—particularly the collapse of the automobile industry in Flint and Detroit—and traced the socioeconomic and political events of the past few decades, I felt I could better comprehend the root causes of deteriorating healthcare in America. Today, I believe I understand why healthcare in America is so expensive and why millions of Americans cannot afford health insurance, leaving them uninsured or underinsured.

Calvin Coolidge once said, *"The business of America is business."* Naturally, over the past three decades, healthcare followed suit, transforming into a commercialized medical-industrial complex that aligned with America's enterprising, capitalistic mindset. Paradoxically, instead of making healthcare cost-effective and affordable, market forces escalated medical expenses to prohibitive levels for many Americans.

As a result, some American industries that provided healthcare benefits to their employees became less competitive compared to their overseas counterparts. General Motors was no exception. The automobile industry began relocating some manufacturing to Mexico while other operations moved to Canada. Many other industries followed suit, with manufacturing jobs going to China and information technology jobs to India.

The standard of living for much of India's middle class improved—ironically, at the expense of America's middle class, which continued to shrink and slide into poverty. As the American economy declined and manufacturing jobs disappeared, unemployment rose. Increasingly, people lost their jobs and their homes. General Motors employees and retirees, who once enjoyed comprehensive healthcare coverage, saw those benefits steadily reduced.

On September 11, 2001, the unthinkable happened. The twin towers of the World Trade Center collapsed into fiery, smoky rubble. The lives of more than three thousand innocent Americans came to an abrupt and tragic end. In response, President Bush went to war in Afghanistan to dismantle Al Qaeda, the group responsible for the attacks on the WTC and the Pentagon. While that conflict was ongoing, he also initiated a second, devastating, and entirely unnecessary war in Iraq.

The shock and awe of relentless bombing caused unimaginable destruction and suffering in Iraq. Meanwhile, there was also shock and awe in America, stemming from the human and economic costs of the war. While the value of the more than 4,000 young soldiers who died in Iraq and the 40,000 who were disabled can never be quantified, the financial toll is measurable. The wars in Afghanistan and Iraq were charged to the national credit card for a staggering $3.1 trillion.

This massive expenditure placed a severe burden on the American economy and contributed significantly to the rising national debt. The economic strain was compounded by another crisis: the bursting of the housing bubble, which had been built on a shaky and immoral foundation. This collapse devastated countless honest Americans who lost their homes and sense of security. The economy spiraled into a deep recession, and millions of people lost their jobs, along with their employer-provided health insurance.

Many middle-class families slipped into poverty, struggling to access even basic healthcare. A few years ago, 60% of Americans had private health insurance, while about 30% relied on Medicare, Medicaid, or Veterans healthcare, leaving 10% uninsured. Today, the numbers are even more disheartening. Seventeen percent of Americans are uninsured, and 50% depend on government-run Medicare and Medicaid.

Curiously, the economic downturn seemed to bypass the CEOs of major corporations, banks, for-profit hospitals, pharmaceutical companies, and insurance firms. They continued to thrive, even as national employment and healthcare conditions worsened.

Yet, politicians in Washington, D.C., appear indifferent to the problem. Many claim that American healthcare is the "best in the world." But I believe they are conflating *"best technology"* with *"best healthcare."* There is a significant difference between the two.

The primary reason healthcare in America continues to deteriorate is that many lawmakers and key players in the medical industry are either unaware or unwilling to confront the cancer that is eating away at American healthcare.

At the core of the American capitalistic ethos is profit. Unfortunately, the pursuit of profit is often unchecked, morphing into a destructive force that corrodes every system it touches. Healthcare is no exception.

*****

Clearly, healthcare in America is a business, and the business of business is profit.

–Anonymous

THE CANCER

The knee was splayed open as the electric saw cut into the top of the tibia, the lower leg bone that forms the knee joint, along with the femur, the thighbone. It's an image I can't forget—the buzzing noise of the saw, the sight of the exposed bone—because the knee belonged to my father. He was undergoing a left knee joint replacement, getting a metallic artificial joint. His osteoarthritis had progressed to the point where the cartilaginous cushion in his knee was completely worn out, leaving bone grinding against bone.

I am a neurosurgeon, not an orthopedic surgeon. My specialty is fixing problems of the brain and spine, not knee or hip joints. But when I saw how my father was limping from pain, even while using a cane to reduce pressure on his knee, I suspected he might need the joint replaced. My suspicions were confirmed when I reviewed his X-rays.

On the day of the surgery, as my father was being wheeled into the operating room, the orthopedic surgeon invited me to watch the operation. For a moment, I hesitated, uncertain if I wanted to witness the blood and bones of my father's knee being cut. What if something went wrong during the surgery? As a surgeon myself, I knew all too well that, despite the safety of modern surgeries, unexpected complications can happen—even death.

How would I feel if something like that occurred?

Despite my concerns, I decided to observe the operation. I changed into surgical scrubs and walked into the operating room. My father had already received spinal anesthesia and was numb from the waist down but fully awake. His knee had been prepped and draped with sterile coverings, one of which extended up to his groin, separating the operative field from the rest of his body.

I walked to the other side of the sterile field and asked my dad how he was feeling. He told me he couldn't feel his legs at all—a sign that the spinal anesthesia was working as intended. Throughout the procedure, I periodically spoke with my dad, who was awake but pain-free, as the surgeon made the skin incision, exposed the bones of the joint, and cut parts of his femur and tibia to prepare for the artificial joint.

The prosthesis was made of a titanium alloy and manufactured by DePuy, a subsidiary of Johnson & Johnson, a prominent American pharmaceutical and medical device company. However, the surgery was being performed in a corporate hospital in Hyderabad, the capital city of my home state of Andhra Pradesh, India. It was just three days before the start of 2012.

Yes, one can undergo state-of-the-art surgeries in India's corporate, for-profit hospitals, performed by surgeons trained in America or Europe, using prosthetic devices also manufactured in America or Europe. The surgeon conducting my father's operation had been trained in England. Thankfully, everything went smoothly, and I was relieved.

When it was time to pay the bill, I reviewed the total expenses and was shocked—not by how expensive it was, but by how affordable it turned out to be. The bill included all pre-surgery tests, four days of hospital care in a private room, the surgeon's fees, the operating room charges, and the imported artificial knee joint. It also covered post-surgery services from neurology and cardiology specialists, as my father had experienced temporary confusion and chest pain after the procedure—both of which he recovered from without issue. Additionally, the bill included 10 days of home physical therapy after discharge, a service typically billed separately in America.

The cost of all this? Less than $8,000.

For context, the average cost of a total knee replacement in the United States is around $55,000. Yet, the $8,000 in India not only covered the same procedure but included significantly more services than would have been covered by the far higher amount in America.

I was astonished. To add to my surprise, the cost even covered my father's admission to the hospital the day before surgery—something that American insurance companies almost never pay for.

I still haven't fully come to terms with the enormous disparity in healthcare costs between India and America for the same procedure performed with comparable quality. Corporate hospitals in India, like their counterparts in America, prioritize their bottom line and aim for profit. Yet, how can we explain the staggering difference in cost—almost five to ten times more in America? The only rational explanation is that healthcare in America is not just commercialized; it is driven by something beyond profit.

My suspicions were confirmed when I read *America's Health Care Crisis Solved* by J. Patrick Rooney and Dan Perrin, who were instrumental in promoting health savings accounts during the George W. Bush administration. In their book, they don't hold back, explaining the primary reason healthcare costs in America have spiraled out of control:

"The problem is greed. The ship has lost its moral rudder. It is awash in greed. The money is too easy and the greed too strong."

Having spent years in private medical practice and witnessing what I have seen around me, I am compelled to agree with their observation.

There you have it—*greed.* Greed is the cancer eating away at and destroying the American healthcare industry.

But who, exactly, is greedy?

Do doctors shoulder all the blame? What about the money-hungry medical malpractice trial lawyers? Or the highly profitable pharmaceutical and medical device manufacturers? How much do the CEOs of hospitals and insurance companies—both for-profit and so-called not-for-profit—pocket as bonuses while patients are driven to bankruptcy by exorbitant insurance premiums and hospital bills?

What about the enterprising private diagnostic centers, nursing homes, and home healthcare companies? How much are they contributing to skyrocketing healthcare costs?

And finally, what about the politicians—the lawmakers responsible for creating a society where affordable, quality healthcare remains out of reach for millions of Americans?

Even patients themselves—do they bear any responsibility for this crisis? These questions are critical as we examine the tangled web of greed within the American healthcare system.

I believe the answer is that players from all facets of the healthcare system share responsibility for driving up costs. Are some doctors ordering unnecessary tests and performing more procedures than required? Are pharmaceutical and medical technology companies inflating the prices of drugs and devices? Are hospitals and insurance companies overcharging patients? Do some patients engage in unhealthy lifestyles that lead to chronic illnesses, resulting in preventable overuse of healthcare services? Are politicians excessively influenced by lobbying from special interest groups, creating laws that prioritize profits over public well-being?

The answer is yes to all of the above.

The Institute of Medicine, part of the National Academy of Sciences and an independent advisor to the government and public, recently published a report that sheds light on this issue. Written by 18 top-tier clinicians, policy experts, and business leaders, the report reveals that the American medical system wastes an estimated $750 billion annually while failing to deliver high-quality care consistently. To put that into perspective, $750 billion is equivalent to the annual cost of health coverage for 150 million workers, the budget of the Department of Defense, or the 2008 bank bailout.

Analyzing the 2009 data, the report highlights the following:

- $210 billion was spent on unnecessary services, such as duplicate tests.

- $130 billion was wasted on inefficiently delivered services, like scans performed in hospitals instead of outpatient centers.
- $75 billion lost to fraud.
- $55 billion was spent on missed prevention opportunities.
- $190 billion was wasted on paperwork and excessive administrative costs.

The only two underlying reasons for these inefficiencies and abuses of healthcare dollars are inefficiency and profit-driven greed.

The corrosive effects of greed permeate the entire spectrum of medical services. I would like to delve deeper into this issue, starting with the role physicians play in escalating healthcare expenses and, consequently, in the deterioration of healthcare in America.

*****

There are three reasons for unnecessary spinal fusions: greed, ignorance, and stupidity. The big problem is greed. I hate to say it, but most neurosurgeons want to do spine surgery because, at this time, it is lucrative.

–Harold D. Portnoy, M.D. Pontiac, MI

HIPPOCRATES WHO?

The patient was wheeled into one of the examination rooms in my office on a stretcher. Just a few days earlier, she had been able to walk—but not anymore. She had experienced neck pain for years and occasional numbness in her hands, but she didn't think much of it. She wasn't the type to see a doctor for intermittent symptoms.

When her arms and legs began to weaken, she attributed it to old age. However, as her symptoms worsened, the numbness in her hands became constant. Her arms and legs grew progressively weaker to the point where she needed a walker, though her grip on it was unsteady. Eventually, her legs became so weak that she couldn't stand, and her arms weakened to the extent that even feeding herself became a challenge.

Finally, realizing the severity of her condition, she sought medical help. Her family doctor immediately recognized the seriousness of her neurological issues and referred her to a neurologist. Eventually, she was referred to my office. By the time she arrived, she had been bedridden for several days, which was why she was brought in on a stretcher.

I examined her on the stretcher, as transferring her onto the examination table was too uncomfortable and difficult. Her medical history and the progression of her symptoms, combined with my physical examination, strongly indicated spinal cord compression in her neck.

An MRI of her cervical spine confirmed the diagnosis. She had severe cervical spondylosis, with significant pressure on both the nerves and spinal cord caused by protruding cartilaginous discs and bone spurs in the cervical spine. The MRI also revealed a white signal within the spinal cord itself, indicating damage to the cord.

She undoubtedly needed surgery, but I wasn't optimistic about her chances of regaining strength, even after the procedure. Once significant damage occurs to the spinal cord, the odds of a complete recovery become slim. The ideal time for surgery would have been before she developed such severe weakness and numbness. At that point, we might have been able to prevent further deterioration. Unfortunately, it was too late for that, but I was determined to give her the best chance possible. Still, I felt deeply saddened by her grim prognosis. Even with surgery, she might never walk again.

While reviewing the rest of her diagnostic tests, I came across one performed by the neurologist that left me seething with anger. It was an Electromyography (EMG) study—a test in which needles are inserted into muscles in the arms and legs, followed by small electric shocks, to diagnose the cause of muscle weakness.

What enraged me was that this test was completely unnecessary. The neurologist could have easily made the diagnosis based on her history and a thorough physical examination. A competent neurologist would have localized the problem to cervical myelopathy in her neck through these basic clinical methods, which would then lead to ordering an MRI to confirm the provisional diagnosis. That's the standard approach any skilled neurologist should follow.

Instead, this doctor inserted needles into nearly every muscle in both her arms and legs. It was not only unnecessary but also painful and distressing for a patient who was already suffering, desperate, and trusting the doctors she turned to for help. Conducting such a test under these circumstances was unethical, morally indefensible, and simply wrong.

I have no doubt the neurologist charged for every needle insertion and electrical stimulation, likely adding up to a significant sum. The only plausible explanation for his decision to perform the test was greed.

Just as I was angry, anyone who understood the motive behind performing such an unnecessary, painful test on this vulnerable patient would feel the same way.

Not all physicians are greedy. Most are conscientious and genuinely care for the well-being of their patients. They strive to do the right thing, avoid causing harm, and refrain from subjecting patients to unnecessary tests or procedures. However, it's not uncommon to encounter some doctors who do otherwise, particularly when they own diagnostic tools within their practices. The more tests they perform, the more they earn. The temptation to prioritize profit over necessity can be difficult to resist.

Examples of such diagnostic tools include equipment for routine colonoscopies, EKGs, echocardiograms, EMGs, X-rays, ultrasounds, CT scans, and MRI machines. Given the fee-for-service model of medicine in America, where revenue from tests forms a substantial part of a physician's income, it's unsurprising that diagnostic tests are often over-utilized. Reimbursement is based on the quantity of care rather than its quality, incentivizing excessive testing.

I recall 1995, the year I began my practice, when managed care was just starting to curb unnecessary testing. That year, the number of coronary angiograms performed dropped dramatically. My first thought was: *Why were so many unnecessary angiograms being done in the first place?*

As physicians, we should take responsibility for policing ourselves, ensuring that only necessary tests and procedures are performed. This would prevent situations where non-medical administrators from insurance companies dictate when a test can or cannot be conducted. Unfortunately, achieving self-policing among physicians is far from easy, especially in today's environment.

As healthcare costs rise, insurance companies and Medicare continue to cut reimbursements for physicians' services. To compensate for this loss of revenue, some practices resort to increasing the number of diagnostics and procedures: more EMGs of arms and legs, more ultrasounds to check for carotid artery narrowing, more coronary angiograms, and even more surgeries with potential lifelong complications—all too often when they are not truly necessary.

I'm not condoning these unnecessary tests or procedures. It's simply a sad reality of the system we're operating within.

Some unnecessary tests are performed because clinical guidelines on their usefulness or appropriateness remain unclear, often due to a lack of sufficient research. Even when evidence accumulates against certain diagnostic or therapeutic practices, it can take nearly a decade for that information to filter into everyday medical practice, shifting the deeply ingrained beliefs and habits of physicians.

For instance, the United States Preventive Services Task Force has recommended against routine screening tests for several common conditions: prostate cancer screening in men over 75 years old, cervical cancer screening in women over 65 years old, and colonoscopies in patients over 75 years old. Despite these guidelines, these tests are still routinely conducted.

The same holds true for certain procedures, such as coronary stent placements, C-sections, and spine surgeries. In a *New York Times* article titled *"Squandering Medicare's Money"* (May 25, 2011), Dr. Rita Redberg—a cardiologist, professor of medicine at the University of California, San Francisco (UCSF), and editor of the *Archives of Internal Medicine*—points out that many unnecessary coronary stents are still being placed. This continues even though clinical trials have shown that medications and lifestyle changes are equally effective for many patients.

Dr. Redberg also highlights that more than 20% of implantable defibrillators are deemed ineffective, yet they are implanted regardless. Each device costs between $50,000 and $100,000, representing a significant financial burden on the healthcare system.

This disconnect between evidence and practice underscores the challenges of reducing unnecessary medical interventions, even in the face of clear recommendations.

As a surgeon, I agree with Dr. Redberg that surgical interventions are often overutilized. For instance, when managed care began limiting the number of C-sections, I wondered why so many deliveries were performed via Caesarean to begin with, when natural deliveries might have been possible.

Being a brain and spine surgeon, I also see firsthand that the United States performs more spine surgeries than any other developed country. Between 1990 and 2001, the number of lumbar fusion surgeries increased by 220% in America. While it's debatable how many of these surgeries are truly necessary, some are clearly performed out of greed.

For example, a spine surgeon in Oregon was barred from operating by the hospital after being accused of performing multiple unnecessary surgeries on the same patients and even billing for surgeries that were never performed. If the allegations are true, this surgeon exemplifies greed at its worst, showing complete disregard for the Hippocratic oath. Subjecting a patient to unnecessary, potentially life-threatening surgery for personal gain is unforgivable.

One alleged factor in his behavior was his involvement in a Physician Owned Distributorship (POD) of spinal implants—devices like screws for stabilizing the spine or artificial joints. In a POD arrangement, a physician bypasses third-party distributors, purchases implants directly from manufacturers, sells them to hospitals, and profits from the markup.

This surgeon reportedly brought patients who had previously undergone spinal instrumentation surgery back into the operating room, removed their existing hardware, and replaced it with implants from his own distributorship. If true, this is highly unethical and immoral.

While some physicians are indeed driven by greed to perform unnecessary interventions, many others are motivated by a different concern: the fear of frivolous lawsuits brought by a different group of greedy individuals—lawyers.

*****

Ambulance chaser (n. *Slang*)

1. **A lawyer who obtains clients by persuading accident victims to sue for damages.**
2. **A lawyer avid for clients.**

AMBULANCE CHASERS

The doctor is alleged to be responsible for the death of a newborn baby. The nurse who administered the sedating barbiturate medication to the infant claims the doctor wrote the order for it. The doctor denies this allegation. A criminal lawsuit against the doctor is currently ongoing. While medical errors are a significant cause of death in many countries, and medical malpractice lawsuits are abundant in America, this case is different. It is the only malpractice case against a physician in an entire country with a population exceeding nine million—Sweden.

When I first heard about this case, I was shocked. Having practiced neurosurgery in America for over sixteen years, I am well acquainted with the medical malpractice climate here. To learn that there is only one medico-legal case against a physician in all of Sweden was astounding. It's a truly incredible statistic.

When Robert, a doctor from the Department of Public Health in Stockholm, told me about the case, the first thought that ran through my mind was, *"How is that even possible?"*

Personal injury lawyers in America are arguably the most aggressive in the world. Billboards along highways urge people to call lawyers if they've experienced complications or undesirable outcomes from medical interventions, devices, or pharmaceuticals. Turn on the TV, and you're almost guaranteed to see commercials advertising massive awards for medical injury claims. And then, of course, there are the ambulance chasers.

The stark contrast between the legal climates in America and Sweden is striking, and it highlights a significant cultural and systemic difference in how medical malpractice is handled.

When I first heard the term *ambulance chaser,* I thought it was a joke. Apparently, it's not. Some lawyers have "connections" with ambulance or emergency-room personnel who notify them when auto accident victims are taken to the ER. These lawyers then approach the injured patients, persuading them to sue for damages.

Recently, I came across a for-profit business that advertises on behalf of personal injury lawyers for auto-accident victims. These lawyers often refer patients to a handpicked group of doctors, physiatrists, pain management specialists, and surgeons. This group tends to determine that the accident was the cause of their patient's pain, particularly chronic back or neck pain.

Some of these surgeons proceed to perform complex spinal instrumentation surgeries for back and neck pain despite knowing the questionable outcomes of such interventions. Worse, they are often aware that some patients are exaggerating or fabricating their pain for monetary gain. Tragically, some of these patients, whether knowingly or unknowingly, risk worsening their condition, developing new pain, or even enduring lifelong complications—all for the sake of financial compensation.

Neurosurgical literature consistently reports that ongoing litigation or attorney involvement is one of the most significant negative predictors of a satisfactory outcome after surgery. It's an unethical scam when medical business entrepreneurs, lawyers, and doctors collaborate to exploit or even create pain, disability, depression, and misery just to secure financial payouts—payouts that often benefit the lawyers far more than the patients. Sadly, this is not an uncommon scenario in America.

The stark contrast in the relative scarcity of active medical lawsuits in Sweden, compared to the United States, piqued my curiosity. I wanted to understand how their system manages to function without ambulance chasers.

Sweden's medico-legal system, shared by other Scandinavian countries, operates under a "no-fault" model. It is designed to care for patients harmed by avoidable risks and complications, defective equipment, incorrect diagnoses, or infections contracted during treatment. The system does not assign blame but focuses solely on providing compensation and care for injured patients.

Nearly 99% of claims are settled by adjustors from medical malpractice insurance companies, funded by doctors collectively through malpractice premiums. There are caps on pain and suffering awards, making settlements more predictable and affordable. This no-fault system is typically faster and less expensive than America's litigation-driven model.

If patients are dissatisfied with their settlement, they can appeal to a nine-member panel. They also have the option to file their case in a judicial court, but this is rare. This rarity explains why ambulance chasers are virtually nonexistent in Sweden.

In contrast to the no-fault system, the American tort system is adversarial. When cases go to jury trials, the process becomes prolonged, stressful, and expensive. Juries often award substantial sums for pain and suffering, but a significant portion of the money doesn't reach the suffering patient. Instead, lawyers frequently benefit disproportionately. Just ask John Edwards if you need an example.

This process is taxing for both patients and doctors. While it's essential to prevent incompetent and negligent doctors from causing harm, many lawsuits filed in America are frivolous or non-meritorious. When conscientious and competent doctors are forced to defend against such lawsuits, they often feel humiliated and depressed. Doctors, by and large, are not psychologically equipped for legal combat.

The merits of the American tort medical malpractice law system are debatable. However, one major unintended consequence is the widespread practice of defensive medicine.

To protect themselves from legal challenges, many doctors order more tests and perform more procedures than necessary. This practice, known as *defensive medicine,* adds significant costs to the healthcare system. Reliable estimates suggest that defensive medicine costs the U.S. as much as $190 billion annually. A recent study of 1,200 orthopedic surgeons revealed that 90% had practiced some form of defensive medicine in the past year. Moreover, 42% of them reported restricting their practices to avoid complex, risky procedures or litigious patients.

Reforming tort medical-malpractice law must be part of any comprehensive healthcare cost-cutting strategy for America. Unfortunately, the political will for such reform has been weak. President Obama stated his desire to increase access to quality healthcare while controlling costs, and he acknowledged the challenges doctors face when constantly worrying about aggressive trial lawyers. Yet, tort reform was not among his priority issues.

President George W. Bush also occasionally mentioned the need for tort reform during his presidency. However, even during the years when the House, Senate, and White House were under Republican control, no significant reform was enacted.

Why is medical malpractice law so difficult to reform?

One plausible reason is the overrepresentation of lawyers in American lawmaking. While lawyers make up only about 6% of professionals in the United States, 45% of members of Congress are lawyers. It's likely that lawyer-legislators hesitate to cut into the revenue streams of their trial-lawyer colleagues, who profit from suing doctors, medical device manufacturers, and pharmaceutical companies.

Speaking of the pharmaceutical industry that is another significant player contributing to America's uncontrollable medical expenses. At a time when increasing numbers of Americans are unable to afford the life-saving drugs they desperately need, this industry continues to enjoy consistent, incredible profits.

*****

Because the US is the only major industrialized nation that does not regulate the prices or profits of drug companies, prescription drugs generally cost 25 to 40 percent more than in other countries. For three out of four elderly Americans, prescription drugs are their biggest expense.

–Elaine Feuer Innocent Casualties

PLATINUM PILLS

He felt like killing himself.

He said he was deeply depressed.

"Suicidal ideation" was the reason Joe Gray was admitted to the hospital for a week and a half.

I met him in Washington, D.C., in October 2011. He was a leader among the Occupy DC protesters marching through Freedom Plaza. When I first saw him, I never would have believed he had once contemplated suicide. He didn't look like someone who would consider taking his own life.

He looked tough. With a shaven head, a groomed beard, and a mustache, he carried an air of resilience. A horseshoe-shaped ring hung from the septum of his nose, resting on his upper lip, while another pierced the upper part of his right ear. Two penny-sized blue rings stretched the lobes of his ears. When he moved his head while talking, the fluttering leaves of a tree behind him were visible through those rings.

After his discharge from the hospital, Joe joined a psychological therapy group. He now takes anti-anxiety medication four times a day. Each pill costs him $6, amounting to $700 for a month's supply and $8,400 per year. That's an enormous amount of money for just one drug to help keep his nerves under control.

When I spoke with him, he was grateful to have been able to afford the healthcare and medication that saved his life. But he was running out of money. He was painfully aware of how the pharmaceutical industry was profiting excessively from his hardships—and those of countless other patients like him.

Joe believed that the drug companies, with their powerful lobby in Washington, D.C., intentionally keep costs high to maximize profits. To them, it didn't matter that many people couldn't afford the pills they needed to stay alive. For PhaRMA, the Pharmaceutical Research and Manufacturers of America, the drugs they produce and sell are, figuratively speaking, worth their weight in gold—or perhaps platinum!

It's no surprise that pharmaceutical companies are the most profitable among all Fortune 500 companies in America, boasting profit margins between 13.5% and 31%, even in a depressed economy.

Despite their staggering profits, these companies remain unwilling to lower drug prices. They claim that high research and development (R&D) costs justify the prices, suggesting that R&D expenses are higher than their marketing budgets. They strive to present themselves as an industry of "researchers in white coats" dedicated to creating life-saving drugs for the benefit of society.

But is that the true picture?

An independent and thorough analysis published in 2008 concluded that the pharmaceutical industry spends twice as much on marketing and advertising as it does on research and development (R&D)—a stark contradiction to the industry's claims.

Moreover, drug companies significantly benefit from basic science research funded by national science and health institutions using public money. Once a drug is developed, a company gains monopoly rights over it, thanks to government patent policies. These patents allow only one company to produce and sell the drug for years after its creation, enabling predatory pricing and exorbitant profit margins that consumers are forced to bear.

These findings are detailed in *"The Cost of Pushing Pills: A New Estimate of Pharmaceutical Promotion Expenditures in the United States,"* authored in 2008 by researchers Marc-André Gagnon, then a

Ph.D. candidate, and Joel Lexchin, M.D., a longtime investigator of pharmaceutical promotion.

According to Gagnon and Lexchin, in 2004, the pharmaceutical industry spent $61,000 on promotion for each of America's 700,000 physicians. This is hardly surprising. If drug companies want doctors to prescribe expensive medications over equally effective and much cheaper alternatives, they need to cultivate favorable relationships with physicians.

Lavish dinners at upscale restaurants, fine wines, and juicy steaks, all arranged by polished and charming drug company representatives, are common tactics to influence prescribing behavior. In 2004 alone, drug companies spent nearly $43 billion on promotions, expecting these investments to yield substantial profits.

However, the frenzy to promote drugs has implications beyond just high costs. In a rush to maximize profits as quickly as possible, drug makers and their researchers may downplay or even hide the dangerous side effects of certain medications.

A glaring example is Vioxx, a drug that was linked to cardiac complications, including heart attacks and strokes. These risks were not adequately disclosed before the drug received FDA approval. Tragically, approximately 60,000 innocent patients died as a result before Vioxx was finally pulled off the market.

While some lawyers profited from lawsuits related to Vioxx, the drug company responsible, Merck, continues to thrive. It remains the third most profitable pharmaceutical company in the United States.

The pharmaceutical industry, or PhaRMA, has both the money and the power to ensure business continues as usual, including paying its CEOs enormous salaries. In 2010, according to *Fierce Pharma,* Bill Weldon, CEO of Johnson & Johnson, earned $28.7 million; Miles White of Abbott earned $25.6 million; Jeffrey Kindler of Pfizer made $24.7 million; and Richard Clark of Merck took home $24.6 million. That's an astonishing amount of money.

The PhaRMA lobby steers public policy and influences lawmakers to craft legislation that guarantees the industry continues to reap exorbitant profits. Although Americans often tout the virtues of competition as a way to lower costs, U.S. law prevents foreign companies from competing in domestic drug manufacturing or importing lower-cost drugs from abroad. The PhaRMA lobby has erected every conceivable barrier to any policy that might threaten its profits.

In 2003, President George W. Bush signed the Medicare Modernization Act with the well-intentioned goal of helping seniors manage their drug costs. However, the act includes a coverage gap, widely known as the "donut hole." Under this provision, coverage ends when a patient's yearly drug costs surpass approximately $2,400 and resumes only after costs exceed about $6,000.

If drug prices were lower, if competition from companies manufacturing at lower costs were allowed, or if Medicare had the authority to leverage its massive purchasing power, the donut hole could have been closed. Yet, PhaRMA ensured the legislation prohibited the Federal government from negotiating discounts with drug companies or creating a formulary that would approve only less expensive yet equally effective drugs.

The pharmaceutical industry's ability to control politicians—like puppets—is nothing short of staggering.

Today, many seniors—people who worked hard throughout their lives, paid their dues, and expected to enjoy peaceful golden years—are forced to go back to work or face starvation just to afford the medications they need. Meanwhile, the pharmaceutical industry continues to lead all American industries in profits. This stark reality points to a fundamental flaw in both the mission and motives of the drug industry and the government that permits the existence of so many drug monopolies.

It's clear that filling the prescription drug donut hole will remain a challenge as long as drug prices remain so exorbitantly high. The pharmaceutical industry is not only greedy but also extraordinarily powerful. However, its profitability is partly rooted in the basic economic principle of supply and demand. As long as people continue to get sick and rely on medications, pharmaceuticals will remain immensely profitable.

One way to counter this is through prevention. People who adopt healthy lifestyles are less likely to develop serious illnesses such as diabetes, high blood pressure, and strokes. By living healthier lives, individuals can significantly reduce their personal medical expenses and collectively contribute to lowering the massive costs of healthcare in America.

A major contributor to the healthcare crisis is obesity, which brings with it a host of related medical costs. The problem of obesity is expanding—both figuratively and literally—and it is an issue that must be acknowledged and addressed without delay.

When I learned just how widespread the obesity epidemic is in America—and how much worse it is projected to become in the near future—I was taken aback. The implications for public health and healthcare costs are staggering.

*****

(If) we stay on the current track, we're going to see unacceptably high rates of obesity and, more importantly, unacceptably high rates of diabetes, heart disease, stroke, obesity-related cancers, and arthritis, that will really place a huge burden on our health care system.

–Jeff Levi, Executive Director Trust for American Health

LIFESTYLE AND LIFE

She was completely anesthetized! A tube into her lungs was connected to a ventilator, which was doing rhythmic breathing for her. Her eyes were taped shut, and a hospital cap covered her hair. A sterile drape separated her face from the operative field. She was having gastric bypass surgery, her last resort to control her obesity. I knew her well. She is a very pleasant and friendly girl who is desperate to lose weight. She had made the drastic choice of bariatric surgery, knowing that one of the potential complications of that surgery could be death.

Still, she felt she had no choice.

I see Jamie in the operating room two or three days a week, not as a patient but as the clerk who answers the phone at the main desk of the OR. She is 36 years old. She talked to me a few days before the surgery. She said that her life was miserable. She had become a recluse because of her weight. She didn't feel like going out with her husband and children. They have a boat, but she couldn't enjoy it. She wouldn't go swimming or camping. Her obesity had also caused her to have high blood pressure and become borderline diabetic. She has tried everything to lose weight. Finally, she decided it was time to do something drastic to lose weight, so she decided to go ahead with the bariatric surgery. It was a life-and-death decision, literally, because the surgery included the risk of possible death, as mentioned earlier. But if she didn't lose weight, she would suffer a slow and gradual deterioration. Her heart, brain, kidneys, and other organ systems could fail over time. Her knee and hip joints would wear out prematurely.

But one thing that she said stayed in my mind. She said she was an emotional eater. Not eating right and not exercising enough were the reasons why she was obese. She blamed her overweight on her own behavior.

Jamie is not alone when it comes to the problem of obesity in America. It is a huge problem, no pun intended, and it is only getting bigger. Twenty years ago, no state in America had obesity rates greater than 15% of the population. Now, according to the U.S. Centers for Disease Control and Prevention (CDC), 34.9% of the adults in Mississippi are obese, and the CDC projects that by 2030, close to two-thirds of people in that state will become obese. The CDC estimates for the whole country in 2030 are also discouraging: 44% of the population will be obese. In thirty-nine states, half of the adults will be obese; in thirteen, 60% will be obese.

These projections suggest an incredible magnitude of obesity-related consequences for health: increased strokes, high blood pressure, heart disease, and arthritis. Equally staggering will be the monetary costs. Elizabeth Landau, in her article *"Health care costs to bulge along with U.S. waistlines"* (CNN.com, September 18, 2012), says that obesity-related healthcare costs are now around $190 billion but are projected to rise to $550 billion by 2030.

Even though the economic cost of obesity can be estimated, the human cost of obesity-related diseases is incalculable. It is difficult to imagine how a stroke, either from a hemorrhage in the brain due to high blood pressure or from a lack of blood supply to the brain from a clogged artery, will devastate a patient and their family for the rest of their lives. A heart attack, even if nonfatal, can have the same kind of devastating impact. If there is one area where the age-old wisdom that "Prevention is better than cure" needs to be remembered and practiced, it is in preventing obesity-related debilitating strokes and heart attacks.

Surprisingly, a healthy lifestyle is not easy to achieve. One might think that eating healthy, exercising a little, and making other prevention-minded choices shouldn't be that hard. But it is! Enter the government. New York bans jumbo-size sodas, and federal law requires food labels to include calorie content. Of course, the companies that profit more when consumers consume more are not going to like the intrusion of government. On the other hand, if we would voluntarily modify our behavior and make healthy choices, then there would be no need for Big Brother to tell us what to do.

One sector of healthcare that appears to be very concerned about the state of obesity in America is the health insurance industry. This might seem paradoxical and, in fact, does represent a recent change of heart by that industry. I'm not sure if the change has come about because Obamacare requires that preventive visits be included in health insurance benefits at no extra cost or because the industry recognizes that preventive healthcare for their enrollees makes good business sense. Prevention means less disease and less money spent on treating disease, resulting in more money saved for the bottom line. United Healthcare, one of the biggest for-profit insurance companies, has been trying to spread the word about the evils of obesity in America by sponsoring surveys and studies.

However, unlike insurance companies, there are many other sectors of the medical-industrial complex that don't benefit from a healthy nation—pharmaceuticals, for example. We know that drug companies prosper because of unhealthy people. The profits of these companies bulge in proportion to the bulge of the waistlines in America. The other sector of the healthcare industry that will make less profit if the health of the nation improves is the medical-device-manufacturing industry. If the Body Mass Index were to decrease by 5% among the obese, not only would we have a healthier population, but also billions of dollars would be saved on healthcare costs. There would be fewer EKGs, echocardiograms, and coronary angiograms to diagnose and fewer stent and pacemaker placements and heart surgeries to manage heart disease. There would be fewer Dopplers, carotid artery stents, and surgeries to discover and open up clogged *carotid* arteries in the neck (which supply blood to the brain) to prevent or treat strokes. There would be fewer hip and knee replacements with artificial metallic or ceramic prostheses for the joints worn out under the weight of obese bodies. All this means less business for the medical device manufacturers.

We have a largely for-profit medical industry, and some of the device manufacturers are not satisfied with the business they already have from an unhealthy population. They subtly encourage doctors to use their medical and surgical-device products and services in patients who may not really need them. It is not at all uncommon to see such overuse and misuse in the world of American healthcare.

Unnecessary surgeries, as well as improperly used devices and technologies, can cause needless problems and pain for patients. They could even be fatal, but these companies don't mind as long as their coffers continue to be filled.

*****

Federal enforcement authorities are focusing on key fraud and abuse issues in the medical device industry - safety-related reporting and fraud risks, kickbacks, device alteration and off-label marketing

–Virginia Gibson US Attorney's Office presentation May 24, 2007

DEADLY DEVICES

Sally couldn't breathe and began to panic. Her breathlessness worsened and turned into gasping. She started to lose awareness and become lethargic. The nurse called for a "code blue," the emergency signal, to get help for respiratory or cardiac arrest. When the code team arrived, they saw the patient's neck severely swollen, and she was cyanotic, blue from lack of oxygen. She was unconscious. The respiratory therapist placed a facemask connected to an oxygen tank with 100% oxygen over the patient's nose and mouth and started squeezing the rubber bag to pump oxygen into the lungs. Unfortunately, it was not enough for the kind of emergency Sally was facing. The patient needed intubation—passing a tube into the lungs and connecting it to a ventilator. The anesthesiologist from the emergency code team attempted to intubate. That was unsuccessful. The neck was too swollen, pushing and compressing the trachea and the windpipe, preventing the tube from passing between the vocal cords into her lungs. Time was running out. If the brain doesn't get oxygen for more than three minutes, parts of it are damaged permanently, and after more than five minutes, further extensive damage will occur. A second attempt was also unsuccessful. There was no choice other than an emergency bedside tracheotomy—stabbing into the trachea with a needle just below the mid part of the neck in the front to allow oxygen into the lungs through a small tube. That small stab wound would later be converted into a tracheostomy by placing and securing a larger tube in the operating room.

That's what happened to Sally. Unfortunately, there was a period of more than five minutes during which her brain didn't receive enough oxygen. She sustained extensive anoxic damage to her brain.

She went into a coma. She was placed on artificial respiration but died a few days later.

A day prior to that tragic event, she was a healthy woman, except that she had neck and arm pain from pinched nerves, a condition called cervical spondylosis. Neck surgery for cervical spondylosis is very common if non-surgical treatments do not relieve the pain. It involves making an incision from the front of the neck and gently dissecting and moving the windpipe and food pipe to the side to reach the front of the spine. Then, the cartilaginous disc between the vertebrae of the spine, protruding backward and pinching the nerve, is removed. Sometimes, bone spurs, also pinching the nerves, are drilled off at the same time. After that, the gap between the vertebrae is bridged with either a simple bone graft or plastic (PEEK) or metal cages filled with bone graft.

Even though complications such as difficulty breathing, difficulty swallowing, nerve injury, or even death are possible, they are rare. The surgery has become routine. The only difference in Sally's surgery was that a new biologic called Infuse, a liquid that contains rtBMP, which stands for recombinant tissue bone morphogenetic protein, was used in the cages to increase the formation of new bone and fuse the two vertebrae together. (A biologic is a product derived from living sources rather than simple chemistry. Vaccines are biologics.)

The FDA approved the use of Infuse in cages as part of lumbar spine (lower back) surgery via an anterior or front approach only. In Sally's case, it was used in her neck surgery as an "off-label" use. Off-label uses are common in medicine. Unfortunately, it was alleged that this use of the BMP in the neck was responsible for the inflammation and swelling that resulted in the compression of the windpipe, eventually causing her death. A lawsuit was filed against the manufacturer of Infuse, Medtronic.

Two more people, who required emergency intervention but fortunately survived, filed similar lawsuits. Their claim was that there was an FDA warning about off-label use. It was further alleged that surgeons conducting the clinical trials "underreported" complications.

The issue of "underreporting" is controversial. The concern is that the huge monetary rewards the spine surgeons received from Medtronic as "consultation fees" during the clinical trials could have biased them from reporting the true extent of complications.

The details of exactly what happened in the testing of Infuse will presumably be settled by the legal cases still being litigated in the courts. However, we know for certain that the company paid many surgeons handsome consultation fees, in some cases hundreds of thousands of dollars, to knowingly use their product off-label. Since such monetary compensation is considered to be a "kickback," which is illegal, a whistleblower lawsuit was filed by the federal government for Medicare fraud against Medtronic as well as many surgeons. The company settled the suit by paying more than $40 million to the government. That is nothing compared to the revenue the company is said to have made selling Infuse—more than $16 billion. That's right. Billions! Not millions of profit. What is a $40 million fine against a $16 BILLION profit? Insignificant!

Money was not the only method the company used to influence the surgeons. They were flown to swank destinations like Miami, Las Vegas, and Cancun and treated to lavish dinners in expensive restaurants. The whistleblowers also alleged that some of the surgeons were taken by the representatives of the company to strip clubs for even more exotic entertainment. These extravagant and expensive promotional practices are not used by Medtronic only; many medical device manufacturing companies follow similar practices.

Of course, innovation, promotion, and advancement of technology are important, but a concern for safety and a responsibility to be truthful about potential complications should outweigh the companies' impulse to pursue fast profits by rushing products to market and expediting their extensive use.

Then, there is the situation where a new technological innovation may be properly tested and shown to be safe and effective, but it may not be more effective than existing technologies, which are often less expensive. Yet, the new technology is marketed aggressively. In this case, how does a manufacturing company get doctors to use the more expensive innovation? The doctors are told that the new technology is state-of-the-art and more effective than whatever is in use already, and then they are lavishly entertained. When it comes to selling modern medical technology, manufacturing companies, just like pharmaceuticals, spend a lot of money on marketing. The companies then mark up the prices of their products to cover all those extra costs and, in this way, still manage to have considerable profits.

A good example of a product with unreasonable pricing is the pedicle screw, used in spinal surgery. It is a metallic screw, usually made of titanium alloy. Each screw sells in America for around $500–$1,000. The same screw costs significantly less in Japan, Europe, Korea, and India. Screws from those countries are not smaller or less strong. They just are not overpriced! The pricing in those countries is regulated. An American sales representative from one of the spine instrumentation companies that manufactures and sells those screws told me that he felt very bad that companies like his ruthlessly overpriced their products. He felt that such price gouging was unethical and shouldn't have any place in the medical field, which is about healing sick people. He told me that the price of the screw is marked up ten to a hundred times more than the manufacturing costs. If a screw actually costs $50 to produce, it may sell for $5,000 in America because there is no regulation or price control. The "free market" rules, and the profit-driven free market is greedy and has questionable ethics. I understand that R&D and logistics have their associated additional costs beyond manufacturing, but other countries deal with the same costs and don't charge as much. When a patient's spine gets screwed in America, their wallet gets screwed, too.

I don't expect any near-term changes in the regulation of medical device manufacturers. Just like other sectors of the medical-industrial complex, they have their connections in the political world of Washington, D.C. In any case, as long as patients, medical insurance companies, the Veterans Administration, worker's compensation, Medicare, and Medicaid keep paying what is charged, the prices will remain unreasonably high.

However, the CEOs of some hospitals have figured out that they can either bargain for prices with medical company representatives (even while not cutting what the hospital charges the patients) or collude with the distributors of the devices to get their share of the inflated pricing.

Not only that, but the sad part is that CEOs of many hospitals encourage as many procedures as possible to be done in their facilities. This is called increasing their "market share" in the community. For the administrators—sorry, Chief Executive Officers—of these hospitals, the more procedures, whether necessary or not, that are done in their institutions, the more profit and bonuses they take home. To these CEOs, patients are customers, and their suffering is simply a matter of business, a matter of dollars and cents.

That brings me to the world of hospitals in America, some of which have transformed themselves from non-profit, mission-oriented institutions devoted to healing the sick into for-profit, greedy, margin-over-mission corporations—a trend that is disturbing.

*****

Florida Hospital simply operated according to standard operating procedures followed by nonprofit hospitals all across the nation. The unwritten rule is to avoid the uninsured when possible and, when not, to gouge them with prices three to five times higher than what others pay. Almost all our hospitals are doing these things

–J Patrick Rooney & Dan Perrin: America's Health Care Crisis Solved

MARGIN OVER MISSION

The chainsaw cut six of the tendons in Steve's left forearm. It was a freak accident. Steve is a landscaper from the suburbs of Detroit. He was cutting the branches of a tree while standing on a ladder. Usually, he has an assistant who steadies the ladder, but the assistant couldn't make it to work that day. Steve thought he could handle the job by himself. He got on the ladder, which was leaning against the tree, and was almost done cutting the branches when the ladder moved, causing him to fall. As he was falling, his outstretched left forearm, attempting to break the fall, landed right on the buzzing chainsaw.

Steve was stunned for a minute. When he realized what had happened and looked at his forearm, he saw blood everywhere. He could actually see the cut muscles and tendons. He was taken to a nearby hospital. A plastic surgeon did a great job of sewing the tendons together. As he lay in the hospital bed after surgery, he started worrying about how he was going to be able to continue working. He needed the full function of both his arms to earn a living as a landscaper.

He was also worried for another reason. Just a few months earlier, he had dropped his health insurance. He had decided that he, his wife, and his two young children were healthy and usually didn't need to visit a doctor. He wanted to put the money he was paying for expensive health insurance premiums into a college fund for his kids. Now, the most unexpected, freakish accident had happened. He worried about the hospital bills that were to come. He had no idea how much they were going to be. He was in for a rude shock.

When he saw the bill for hospital charges, he couldn't believe the number. He thought it must be a mistake: The hospital charges were $42,000.

There was no way he could come up with that much money to pay the bill. He called the hospital, pleading for mercy. Could they reduce the amount some? The hospital didn't show any mercy. In fact, it was ruthless. Steve was told that the hospital would place a lien on his house if he didn't pay in full. He felt helpless. He had no idea what he could do. Then, by chance, he happened to hear about "the billing lady." Her job is to dissect hospital bills and show the hospital that there are unnecessary and inflated charges, as well as charges for procedures that were not done. That was what she did with Steve's bill. Steve was charged for more than the actual number of tendons repaired. When all the mistakes and overpricing were uncovered and the negotiations with the hospital were complete, Steve paid a total of $7,400 instead of the original $42,000.

In their book *America's Health Care Crisis Solved*, Patrick Rooney and Dan Perrin describe how hospitals charge and collect more money from the uninsured than they have agreed to accept from the insurance companies. Hospitals never tell innocent patients that "billed charges" and "accepted payments" are not synonymous, and usually, there is a huge difference between the two.

I have seen nonprofit hospitals that have no qualms or conscience about bleeding the uninsured who are faced with a medical emergency. Rooney and Perrin also point out that even Christian charitable hospitals, which are supposed to be about helping the poor, the needy, and the sick, are not immune to these greedy practices: "No religious denomination seems to have clean hands in the matter. The Catholic Church is making more money off of this than anyone because it happens to operate more nonprofit hospitals than anyone. As Catholics who someday stand to account before Christ, this bothers us. Our hope is to hear Him say, 'Well done, thou good and faithful servant,' not 'depart from me, I never knew you.' Jesus would not tolerate 'Christian' hospitals that plead for mercy from the government to get generous tax relief and then turn around and seize the Rodney Vegas of this world by the throat, demanding payment in full when the money isn't there." (The case of Rodney Vega is featured in their book.)

This transformation of service-oriented hospitals into profit-oriented hospitals didn't happen by accident. It was a systematic infiltration of the institutions by money-hungry CEOs with commercial-enterprise thinking. The hospitals became corporations, and the administrators became CEOs. "Margin over mission" triumphed. With the changeover of hospitals to for-profit status and the not-for-profit hospitals behaving exactly like for-profit hospitals, healthcare costs skyrocketed. Hospital charges are now the biggest expense for Medicare (31%) and nongovernmental health insurance companies. At the same time, hospital CEOs are making unbelievable salaries. According to *Becker's Hospital Review* (September 04, 2012), the average base salary for hospital CEOs is $320,486, but many get a lot more when bonuses are included, sometimes millions more.

To understand what a scam these enormous "not-for-profit hospital" salaries are, remember that the CEOs didn't risk their own money to build hospitals. Most nonprofit hospitals are built with community funds. These hospitals' unpaid bills are written off as expenses, and their nonprofit status shelters them from taxes. Since there are no shareholders to whom profits have to be distributed, the CEOs are awarded incredible bonuses.

The CEO of a hospital is not going to complain about their excessive salary so long as the doctors are okay with it and the members of the board of the hospital forget their responsibility for appropriate oversight. These board members seem to forget the definition of "nonprofit." The law states that no person or corporation can make a profit from a nonprofit institution. If there is excess money after expenses, it must be spent on the institution and the community; for example, the hospital could reduce its charges to patients.

Unfortunately, most boards do not seem to understand (or choose to ignore) the philosophy and principles of nonprofits. This lack of oversight emboldens CEOs to be ruthless in the name of "good business practices." They cut the salaries and pensions of the hard-working nurses and ancillary medical and non-medical employees. They bust the nurses' unions. They don't pay the doctors their due compensation for taking emergency calls and threaten doctors who bring attention to the issue that their privileges will be taken away. They bend existing hospital bylaws or create new ones through medical executive committees to circumvent the bylaw process and advance their profits. They do this with the help of some "yes men" doctors on medical executive committees. These collaborators fail to represent the needs and concerns of the doctors and instead act to enable the agenda of the administrations, who in turn use their power to reward the turncoats. The CEOs put business directors on quality-assurance committees to protect incompetent doctors who are their lackeys. They champion the bottom line at the expense of patient safety. Trust me! I am speaking from personal experience. I have seen this with my own eyes.

In the name of efficiency, the CEOs force device manufacturers to offer lower prices, which they don't pass along to patients. Some CEOs even collude with the distributors of medical instrumentation to split the excess profits generated by charging too much for the devices. In California, one hospital CEO was alleged to have partnered with a convicted criminal in creating a spinal instrumentation distributorship that milked millions of dollars off of Workmen's Compensation funds. In another recent case, a distributor was hired by a hospital as a consultant, and spinal surgery revenues went from $3 million to $65 million in just three years. In some other cases, hospital CEOs created ancillary business enterprises owned by their relatives. I guess nepotism is not dead in the hospital industry.

As if all these legal but unethical practices are not sufficient to make profits, some CEOs resort to fraud, like cheating Medicare, which, I think, is very common, and the amounts to which it is defrauded are shocking. A prime example is the case of Rick Scott's hospital conglomerate, Columbia-HCA. Rick Scott was a lawyer specializing in hospital-corporate law. The story goes that he used his own money to leverage a loan that allowed him to purchase two hospitals that were in financial distress in Austin, Texas. He turned them around and bought more hospitals, forming the multi-hospital company Columbia. Eventually, Columbia purchased another multi-hospital company to form the bigger conglomerate, Columbia-HCA, which changed the skyline of Nashville with its shiny skyscrapers. In 1999, the federal government sued Columbia-HCA and fined it $1.7 billion for Medicare fraud. That simply is sickening. No wonder the company grew so big and so fast. I am not sure if any hospital company can grow that fast doing honest business. As if the medical costs of Medicare are not high enough already, these hospitals have made the problem worse by abusing and defrauding taxpayer-funded Medicare, almost bankrupting it.

So, was Rick Scott convicted of a crime and punished? No! As the rumor goes, the board of the company relieved him of his CEO duties and awarded him $100 million. Here's the kicker! Apparently, he spent $40 million of his own money and became the Republican governor of Florida. Now, he wants to transform state-run Medicaid into a private enterprise business of small strip mall walk-in clinics. The word, which may or may not be true, is that his wife may be the owner of the company.

As nauseating as some of these stories of hospital greed are, at least no lives are directly at stake because of denied care. However, when private health insurance companies scam their customers with "denial of care" ploys, patients die as a consequence.

No wonder some of the executive committees of these private commercial insurance companies are called death panels.

*****

Many of them (private health insurance company CEOs) aren't discovering drugs or treating patients. They're middlemen who process the paperwork, fill the pill bottles, and otherwise connect the pieces of a $2 trillion industry.

–Dave Zweifel

REAL DEATH PANELS

My brother was a business owner of a restaurant that he ran with his wife, Marie. In September 2004, he was diagnosed with Stage IV Non-Hodgkin's Lymphoma. In the midst of his chemo treatments, Otto received a phone call and a letter stating his insurance was canceled due to a "material failure to disclose." Apparently, in 2000, his doctor had done a CT scan, which showed an aneurysm and gallstones. My brother was never told of either one of these conditions, nor was he ever treated for them, and he never reported any symptoms for them either. After months of preparation, his stem cell transplant could not be scheduled. My brother's hope of being a cancer survivor was dashed.

That was the testimony of Peggy Raddatz before the U.S. House of Representatives Energy and Commerce Subcommittee on Oversight and Investigations on July 27, 2009.

Stories like that are not uncommon in America. Many patients have died because either cancer treatments, liver transplantation, or other life-saving procedures were unfairly denied by insurance companies. These companies show no pity, even for children. Denial of healthcare, where patients expect to receive covered benefits but those benefits are withheld, is one of the common ways that for-profit commercial insurance companies amass profits.

The practice is called "rescission." Insurance companies will terminate the insurance policies when they don't want to pay for expensive procedures, using the excuse of any unrelated "preexisting conditions." It makes no difference that a patient was not aware of a condition or that the condition was minor or unrelated to the current illness. Insurance companies can also revoke coverage for the entire family if one member fails to disclose any medical condition. The patients lose their healthcare coverage when they need it the most. Recently, a congressional investigation found that three large insurers saved $300 million using this trick. The companies encourage their employees to comb through a patient's medical records and the family's medical records, looking for the tiniest "preexisting condition," like, say, a yeast infection, so that they can revoke the coverage for, say, cancer treatments. These companies are merciless when it comes to profits.

At a "Healthcare Now" rally, a protester's sign expressed this very serious problem of underhanded rescission with cheeky humor: "Private insurance is like a hospital gown; chances are your ass is not covered."

The greed of health insurance companies clouds whatever sense of fairness or mercy their employees might have as individuals. Wendell Potter, who was the senior vice president of public relations for CIGNA, finally had a change of heart and quit. In his book *Deadly Spin*, he explains the corporate PR and the distortion and fear manufactured by America's health insurance industry. He should know because he wrote the talking points to deflect the growing public anger toward CEOs of insurance companies that deny care and make millions in profits, awarding huge bonuses to themselves. Mr. Potter notes in his book that he has witnessed the insurance CEOs flying in private jets and eating on gold-plated china. It's impossible not to get upset imagining CEOs showering themselves with fortunes and living in luxury while patients and family members are pleading for help to cover the medical procedures necessary to save their own lives or the lives of their loved ones.

The salaries and bonuses the CEOs receive are unbelievable. Let me give you an example. Stephen J. Hempsley, CEO of UnitedHealth Group, a commercial health insurance carrier, received $106 million in salary and stock options in 2009. His salary underscores the irony of the following statement he made about healthcare in America: "Today, the American people are questioning whether or not we receive fair value for the $2.6 trillion we, as a society, are expecting to spend this year on our healthcare system. The vast majority, including those of us at UnitedHealth Group, believe the answer is 'No.'"

I have a feeling some, if not all, of these executives, know that they are a part of the problem, but they don't do much to make healthcare less expensive and reasonable. The insurance industry, as a group, had their salaries and bonuses go up 167%, while at the same time, the average American's wages went up only 2%. With companies making so much profit, the right thing for them to do is decrease the cost of their premiums, but executives have no motivation to do this as long as their salaries, bonuses, and stock options are high. The CEOs of some of the other insurance giants—Cigna, Aetna, Humana, and WellPoint—received between $10 million and $18 million in that year. No wonder the compensation for healthcare CEOs is 40% higher than the average compensation for all other S&P 500 companies.

The worst part of this whole system is that insurance companies are just go-betweens. They take money from the enrollees and pay the doctors and hospitals, keeping 15% to 30% as "administrative fees." These companies do not improve the health of the patients. I pay more than $22,000 per year for my and my family's insurance premiums. Not once have I received anything from my insurance company that actually improved my health or well-being. Insurance executives get paid disproportionately high compensation when compared to the value they add to healthcare delivery.

Another trick of these predatory companies is to sell coverage only to ultra-healthy people. If there is any "pre-existing condition," coverage is either denied or premiums increased. In 45 states of the country, such discrimination is allowed, making 12.6 million people unable to obtain any insurance. In nine states, being a victim of domestic violence constitutes a pre-existing condition.

Many of my own patients have had their coverage dropped (and/or benefits denied) the moment they are diagnosed with early diabetes or heart disease. These insurance companies deny needed medical help that could treat disease or ill health in the beginning so that the problems will not become debilitating chronic illnesses. Consider Mary's story.

She had back pain for a few months. I examined her in my office when she came for a consultation. Fortunately, she did not have any symptoms or test results that suggested nerve compression. I looked at the MRI. She didn't have any rupture or degeneration of the cartilage cushions (discs) between the vertebrae of the lumbar (lower back) spine. Her back pain was most likely from her lower back muscles. This situation is very common. Approximately 75% of Americans will have at least one episode of back pain in their lifetimes. Most of them don't need surgery because 80% of them get better with a short course of anti-inflammatory or narcotic medication and physical therapy. That's exactly what she needed, and that was what my treatment plan was going to be.

Since I perform brain as well as spine surgery, I do see many patients like Mary with back pain, many of whom don't need surgery. When I recommended physical therapy to her, she said she couldn't afford it. She had insurance with a managed care company, which charged her $30 for every physical therapy visit. Usually, a patient with Mary's condition needs at least twelve visits, and that would cost her $360 in addition to the premium she was paying for her insurance. That was too much for her.

I gave her a back-care book and told her to follow the precautions and exercises mentioned in the book. If this home treatment isn't successful, she may not have a choice other than to spend some money on physical therapy. If acute back pain is not treated appropriately in the beginning, it can become chronic back pain. With the continued denial of necessary physical therapy, chronic back pain can become a chronic disability. The patient becomes disabled in more ways than one: physically, psychologically, socially, and financially. Sometimes, these patients come to depend on narcotic medication to control the pain. It can ruin their lives and the lives of their loved ones.

The paradox of these insurance policy regulations is that they can cost the companies more in the long run by allowing minor problems to become major. But then, most insurance companies don't pay for visits to doctors for prevention, which would help in preventing or taking proper early care of high blood pressure, diabetes, heart disease, obesity, or strokes. They are about to drop the coverage if there are early signs of any of these problems. That is a very common tactic, and it is being used more and more. What's incredible is that Mary had insurance and paid her premiums regularly, but she still didn't get the coverage she needed.

Healthcare insurance company premiums have skyrocketed by more than 113% since 2001, and so have the companies' profits. Most Americans don't want a government-provided healthcare option because they believe in free-market capitalism and competition. They are expecting their medical problems to be taken care of by their insurance companies. Good luck! They will get a wake-up call when they get sick, especially if it is a serious illness. Many will then realize they didn't get enough coverage for all the money they paid to the insurance companies through the years. Their premiums will go up further while their coverage shrinks.

Of course, they also face the real danger that they may get dropped from their insurance coverage altogether. That has already been the fate of many. In Flint, where I practice, many GM retirees damaged their backs by repetitive bending, twisting, and lifting while standing on concrete for hours each day for many years. I see a lot of them in my office. Their spines have degenerated from all that hard work, an ungrateful and punishing reward for what they had to endure, making the automobile industry prosperous. But that prosperity disappeared in the late twentieth century and the beginning of this century. Rising healthcare costs were one of the forces that broke the backbone of that once-upon-a-time mighty industry. The automobile jobs were outsourced to Canada and Mexico, as many of us already know. GM does not have to pay healthcare benefits for Canadian autoworkers because they are covered by a national health system, whereas Mexican labor is a lot cheaper than American labor. GM retirees who were counting on healthcare coverage during their golden years have had to think about going to work again, as alluded to before, because their medical insurance benefits have been cut, and they simply can't afford their medical expenses.

The sad part of unaffordable healthcare costs in America is that medical illness is the number one cause of personal bankruptcies, and more than 70% of the people who were forced to declare bankruptcy had insurance. The morally bankrupt insurance companies and the medical-industrial complex as a whole are bankrupting the nation and destroying the lives of millions. One day, my eleven-year-old boy and I were watching fish, jellyfish, and sharks in an aquarium. I was reminded of the medical industry. The patients are like jellyfish. Most doctors are conscientious small fish, even though there are a few small unethical doctor sharks. The so-called nonprofit (but really for-profit) hospital CEOs are big sharks, and pharmaceutical company executives are bigger sharks. The biggest predator sharks are the insurance CEOs who deny healthcare coverage, knowing that patients will die from their unethical decisions. No wonder many feel that the executive committees of some of the insurance companies that come up with these inhumane policies are the real death panels.

Can anybody stop the uncontrolled greed of these so-called free-market, enterprising, selfish companies? Where are the laws and lawmakers who are supposed to be overseeing and protecting the public? Laws could discourage criminal gouging and punish it when it happens, but we don't have such laws.

Is it possible that the laws and lawmakers are a major part of the problem?

*****

You take millions from the insurance industries, HMOs, and pharmaceutical companies and deny the people a voice! Single payer national healthcare is what this country needs. What kind of democracy is this?

–Single-payer advocate at protest during Senate hearing on healthcare reform

SENATORS FOR SALE

On May 5, 2009, the Senate Finance Committee held a hearing on healthcare chaired by Senator Max Baucus (D) from Montana. The committee welcomed "invited stakeholders," including representatives of private insurance companies and hospital associations. Some stakeholders, however, were not invited but showed up anyway. These individuals were not representing any large for-profit corporations; they didn't have money or power. They were not allowed to sit at the table and be part of the hearing like the invited guests, who were scheduled to read prepared statements. These "uninvited stakeholders" had to sit with the audience, but they were determined not to let the senators ignore them. They were intent on questioning the committee as to why neither a single-payer nor a public option was being discussed as part of healthcare reform.

One questioner didn't wait for permission: "So let me get this straight. You have fifteen seats at the table and not one for single-payer? Why is that?"

Senator Baucus banged his gavel for order and called the meeting to recess until police escorted the man out. Immediately, another man in the audience stood up: "It's only when people who are living in the park and people who are living on Park Avenue have the same healthcare that everybody will have high-quality healthcare. Single-payer now!" He, too, was escorted out. There were others, Katie Robbins and Dr. Margaret Flowers among them, who stood up and made similar statements to those who were escorted out. All of them were removed from the room by police. This led Senator Baucus to joke, "We need more police."

Should the fight for access to affordable, universal healthcare be a joke to politicians who are supposed to be serving and protecting the citizens who elected them? Lack of health insurance is not a joke; in fact, it is a matter of life and death for citizens without the financial means to afford decent healthcare. The protesters felt that the senators were not representing the interests of the average citizen but, instead, were pandering to the needs of powerful and wealthy special interests, like the commercial private health insurance companies, who view "single payer" or a public option as their nemesis.

Who were these protesters, anyway?

They represented two organizations—PNHP (Physicians for a National Health Program) and Healthcare-NOW—that have been championing a universal single-payer healthcare system for all Americans. These organizations are upset that they are not being included in the debate that is reforming and transforming healthcare delivery in America. They believe that for-profit enterprises, especially commercial health insurance companies, have profited enormously at the expense of many productive Americans while not operating in good faith to improve the health of the nation. These companies have unfairly denied care and jacked up healthcare costs, causing many citizens suffering from serious illness to go into personal bankruptcy. The unethical practices and greed of these companies are partly responsible for the fact that forty-eight million Americans have no health insurance and don't get the medical help they need.

PNHP and Healthcare-NOW believe that for-profit insurance companies will not cover the medical needs of the poor and the sick because such coverage is not profitable. They also believe the solution to the problem is a publicly funded single-payer system or, at least, a public option that competes with private, for-profit commercial insurance companies.

In a single-payer system, there is no multitude of profit-driven private insurance companies. Citizens pay into the system, usually through taxes, and their healthcare expenses are covered by that single entity. Where this kind of system occurs in the world (for example,

Britain, Canada, Sweden, Finland), it is usually publicly funded, but such a system could be funded publicly, privately, or through a combination of the two. One thing is common to all single-payer systems: there are no greedy, highly profitable private insurance companies.

An alternative to a single-payer system is "the public option." This allows for the creation of a government-run health insurance agency to which any citizen would be allowed to subscribe. If the public option is implemented, private insurance companies would continue to operate but would have to compete with government-run agencies. The public option, like Medicare, would be not-for-profit and would be less expensive in terms of competition with commercial interests. The public option has been proposed as being more politically palatable than a single-payer system, but powerful special interests oppose both.

Commercial insurance companies hate both the single-payer option and the public option. It is understandable that they don't want the proponents of these alternatives to have their voices heard during Senate hearings. The special interests will do anything to deny these options to the American people, including buying lawmakers and paying off senators and congressional house representatives to create laws that benefit commercial profits. Of course, they call it lobbying, which ought to stand for "legal robbing." I wonder what the health industry had to pay Mr. Baucus for his power and influence to make sure the public option was off the table.

One-and-a-half million dollars!

According to *Bill Moyers's Journal*, that is the amount of money received by Senator Baucus from the healthcare industry, which, in the few months leading up to the passing of the healthcare reform act, spent $380 million to lobby lawmakers for advertising and campaign contributions.

Mr. Baucus said he "saw a lot to like" in two proposed public options, but he voted against them anyway. Why? Bill Moyers provided a succinct insight in his *Bill Moyers Journal* (PBS, October 9, 2009). In a video clip of the Senate healthcare hearings, Mr. Moyers pointed out Liz Fowler sitting behind Mr. Baucus. She used to work for WellPoint, the largest health insurer in the country, but now she is working with the Senate Finance Committee—the same committee that has the power to give her old employers "exactly what they want: higher profits and no competition from alternative non-profit coverage that could lower costs and premiums." Moyers went on to explain that Fowler replaced Michelle Easton, who was the top health advisor for Senator Baucus. Easton left Baucus's staff to join WellPoint as a lobbyist. The halls of power in America have revolving doors to accommodate "lobbyist out, lobbyist in."

According to Moyers, the health industry alone has six lobbyists for every congressman, and 500 of the lobbyists were previous congressional staff members. The connections the lobbyists have with the lawmakers, made while the lobbyists were staff members, give them access that no average citizen can have. Free-spending, for-profit healthcare companies benefit lawmakers, lobbyists, and special interests at the expense of the rest of the citizens, who end up being the losers.

What is maddening about this blatant bribery of legislators is that it happens in broad daylight. The only outrage came from the few in the hearing who yelled, "What kind of democracy is this?" before being whisked away by the police.

Once all the ruckus and commotion settled down, Senator Baucus said, "Our plan does not include a public option." Why am I not surprised?

Lobbying undermines the fundamental principles of democracy, and it's a shame the public accepts it with so little protest. The power of "one citizen, one vote" is no match for the power of "one corporation, millions of dollars." There is not much bipartisan consensus in Congress these days, but there is plenty of bipartisan succumbing to special interests.

The abuse of lobbying to the point of bribery is the reason why Senator Baucus says he does not have enough votes to pass a public option. The proponents of such an option can't cough up enough campaign contributions to have any political influence.

Some very influential politicians have lied about the popularity of public options. A majority of Americans support public healthcare options, but John Boehner, Speaker of the House, says he has not heard from a single American who wants a public option. Boehner has said that the public option is as unpalatable as "a garlic milkshake." To test the truth of this statement, a young freelance journalist/filmmaker went to Boehner's district in Ohio to see what people really thought. He found many citizens there publicly advocating healthcare for all, either via a public option or a single-payer system. Speaker Boehner may choose to ignore these "Americans," but he cannot truly be unaware that they exist.

Private insurance companies are not the only corporations that have power over politicians. Every large player in the healthcare industry—including pharmaceuticals, hospitals, doctors, and device manufacturers—has their own lobbyists. Every industry—not just healthcare—understands that money buys political influence in America. Rich special interests pay for lobbying and thereby become wealthier. It is a survival-of-the-fattest-wallet political jungle out there, with many very hungry, predatory beasts.

Healthcare in America is in a pathetic state. It is uncoordinated, highly commercialized, and profit-driven, guided by greed and perpetuated by a corrupt political system. It also costs too much—close to $3 trillion. Half of that amount goes for private commercial insurance and includes out-of-pocket expenses by patients. The other half is borne by government funding, including Medicare, Medicaid, the Veterans Administration, the Children's Health Insurance Program (CHIP), and Tricare (for soldiers and their families).

The highest-cost subsector of the entire industry is hospitals, which account for $900 billion, 31% of the total cost of healthcare in America.

Can anybody fix or improve our current moribund healthcare system?

*****

History is made when a leader steps up, stays true to his values, and charts a fundamentally different course for the country. History is made when a leader's passion - passion - is matched with principle to set a new course. Well, ladies and gentlemen, Mr. President (Barack Obama), you are that leader.

–Vice President Joe Biden signing ceremony for the Patient Protection and Affordable Care Act, March 23, 2010

OBAMACARE

It was a historic day in America. Some say it may rank with the historic days when FDR signed the Social Security Act and Lyndon Johnson signed the Medicare Act. What made that day so significant? Healthcare for every American was first proposed close to a century ago; finally, there is a possibility that it will become a reality. The vice president emphasized Obama's accomplishments:

"Mr. President, you've done what generations of not just ordinary but great men and women have attempted to do. Republicans, as well as Democrats, have tried before. Everybody knows the story, starting with Teddy Roosevelt. They've tried. They were real bold leaders. But, Mr. President, they fell short. You have turned, Mr. President, the right of every American to have access to decent healthcare into reality for the first time in American history."

Bringing healthcare to every American has not been an easy task. During the Clinton presidency, when Hillary Clinton was entrusted with leading the creation of a universal healthcare system, her ideas were smashed even before they came out of the closed-door meetings. The forces opposing universal healthcare, or more government involvement in healthcare, have been very powerful.

In the 1930s and the 1950s, FDR and Truman had a taste of that opposition during their presidencies, even when they were trying only to provide health insurance to seniors and people experiencing poverty. In fact, before FDR, concerned citizens tried many times to organize universal healthcare, but they were always thwarted.

Many who have some understanding of the evolution of healthcare in America know that associations of doctors in America made sure universal healthcare wouldn't happen. They also opposed the idea of Medicare when it was proposed by FDR, Truman, and Johnson.

President Obama decided that he better talk to doctors before championing any legislation expanding access to healthcare. He went to the American Medical Association in 2009. During his address, he said, "My signature is not enough. I need your help." He wanted AMA approval, and he got it—barely. Obamacare was accepted by the AMA with 51% Yes and 49% No! In the end, it didn't matter much whether the AMA approved or not because the bill was passed in Congress and signed by the president.

Doctors think that they have the power to significantly affect the political process on matters of healthcare, but they don't. The wheelers and dealers in DC don't care whether doctors are on board or not. Doctors lost most of their political influence when they opposed Medicare but, at the same time, didn't try to assume any healthcare delivery leadership role. The private-business entrepreneurs of commercial health insurance, hospitals, pharmaceuticals, and device manufacturing quietly filled that leadership void. These business interests influence Congress to pass the laws that benefit them. Doctors today have neither the cohesiveness nor the coffers to have any say in the evolution of healthcare delivery in this country. I guess Obama was just being nice to the doctors. He knows he needs to be nicer to another group that is more important for healthcare reform: the congressmen and congresswomen. He must have realized their importance as soon as he became president and started the process of bringing affordable, universal healthcare to all Americans. We can see this by looking at the shift in his approach to achieving universal healthcare from the time he was an Illinois senator to the time he signed Obamacare.

President Obama is a single-payer proponent at heart. He said it himself when he was an Illinois congressman before becoming a U.S. senator. There is a YouTube clip to prove it. When he got elected to the U.S. Senate, he quickly became aware of the politics that would make it very difficult to realize single-payer universal healthcare in

America. After all, the words "single-payer" and "universal healthcare" are associated with socialism and communism in the minds of many Americans and are, therefore, taboo in capitalist America. More importantly, they would kill commercial insurance enterprises.

Single-payer and universal healthcare are for the "evil" European countries. They elicit a negative, nauseating, visceral reaction, especially in Republican senators like Orrin Hatch. To him, any role of government to improve access to healthcare for the many uninsured Americans amounts to the Europeanization of America, which he vehemently opposes! Besides, a single-payer system means the death of commercial health insurance companies that could be financing the re-election campaigns of politicians like Mr. Hatch. I wouldn't be surprised if it's true that the hospital associations and pharmaceuticals joined in the quiet-resistance movement against any government-run or controlled healthcare delivery options. They must have realized that they would be next on the "government control" chopping block.

Because of the power of these special interests over the politicians, Obama knew there were not enough votes for a single-payer system. He downgraded his ambition from single-payer to the "public option," which would not kill commercial health insurance but would merely be a competitor with it. He clearly said during his address to the AMA in 2009 that a public option had to be part of healthcare reform. He didn't realize what a threat that would be to the survival of non-governmental health insurance companies.

These companies made sure that there weren't going to be enough votes for the public option either. It was never even put on the table by Senator Max Baucus, who was entrusted by President Obama to come up with the sixty-vote majority needed to pass his healthcare reform. Senator Baucus made it happen by excluding both the single-payer and public options from Obamacare. The president must have reconciled himself to "something is better than nothing" when it came to healthcare reform. After all, Obamacare was going to be his signature bill, something he had promised during his campaign for the presidency. Thus, Obamacare was born without a single-payer or a public option.

Many say that Obama didn't go far enough with the reform. I agree with that, but Obamacare is a step in the right direction, hard enough to achieve in capitalist America. It does have some good aspects to it. The president highlighted those prior to signing the bill, the Patient Protection and Affordable Care Act (PPACA), also known as Obamacare.

"The bill I'm signing will set in motion reforms that generations of Americans have fought for and marched for and hungered to see. It will take four years to implement many of these reforms fully because we need to implement them responsibly. We need to get this right. But a host of desperately needed reforms will take effect right away."

He enumerated them one by one:

"This year, we'll start offering tax credits to about 4 million small businessmen and women to help them cover the cost of insurance for their employees."

"This year, tens of thousands of uninsured Americans with preexisting conditions, and the parents of children who have a preexisting condition, will finally be able to purchase the coverage they need. That happens this year."

Hopefully, that will increase access to people who are willing to pay the premiums but were denied insurance under the guise of "pre-existing conditions" because insurance companies considered those people potentially less profitable.

"This year, insurance companies will no longer be able to drop people's coverage when they get sick. They won't be able to place lifetime limits or restrictive annual limits on the amount of care they can receive."

That sure is a great thing, and hopefully, it will put a stop to cutting off medical care when patients need it desperately.

"This year, all new insurance plans will be required to offer free preventive care."

Finally, somebody is trying to practice the age-old adage: "Prevention is better than cure."

"And this year, young adults will be able to stay on their parents' policies until they're 26 years old. That happens this year."

That is true. I have personally met young adults who are out of college but still unemployed and who were very happy to be able to stay on their parent's policy. I have even heard them give a "shout-out" to Obama.

"And this year, seniors who fall in the coverage gap known as the doughnut hole will start getting some help. They'll receive $250 to help pay for prescriptions, and that will, over time, fill in the doughnut hole. And I want seniors to know, despite what some have said, these reforms will not cut your guaranteed benefits. In fact, under this law, Americans on Medicare will receive free preventive care without co-payments or deductibles. That begins this year."

The president's words are important because seniors are being told by many Republicans that Medicare is going to be insolvent and their benefits are going to be cut because of Obamacare.

"Once this reform is implemented, health insurance exchanges will be created—a competitive marketplace where uninsured people and small businesses will finally be able to purchase affordable, quality insurance. They will be able to be part of a big pool and get the same good deal that members of Congress get. That's what's going to happen under this reform. And when this exchange is up and running, millions of people will get tax breaks to help them afford coverage, which represents the largest middle-class tax cut for healthcare in history. That's what this reform is about."

The nonpartisan Congressional Budget Office and the Joint Committee on Taxation say the PPACA gives $828 billion in tax cuts and $588 billion to middle-class taxpayers to help cover their insurance needs.

This legislation will also lower costs for families, businesses, and the federal government, reducing our deficit by over $1 trillion in the next two decades. It is paid for. It is fiscally responsible. And it will help lift a decades-long drag on our economy."

One element of the new law is to create pioneer Accountable Care Organizations. These are designed to help cut Medicare expenses by making it more efficient and by paying doctors and hospitals for better care, not more care. We will have to wait to see how this works out.

Then, the president did what every politician does: praise Americans and the lawmakers for their achievements.

"That our generation is able to succeed in passing this reform is a testament to the persistence—and the character—of the American people, who championed this cause; who mobilized; who organized; who believed that people who love this country can change it. And we have now just enshrined, as soon as I sign this bill, the core principle that everybody should have some basic security when it comes to their healthcare. And it is an extraordinary achievement that has happened because of all of you and all the advocates all across the country."

Then, he sat down to sign the bill. After signing, he said, to thundering applause from the audience, which included Nancy Pelosi, Harry Reid, and many other congressmen and congresswomen, as well as some non-politician American citizens, "We are done."

Wow! Wow! Hold your horses, Mr. President. That's a bold statement. Are we really done? I hope you meant you were done with signing the bill and not with the task of realizing universal, affordable healthcare for all Americans. Will Obamacare ensure access to quality healthcare for all Americans? Many don't think it went far enough to achieve that, but, as I said earlier, it is a step in the right direction. President Obama should be given credit for risking his political future and sticking to his principles and ideology.

The million-dollar question is: Will Obamacare survive? Before the ink of the president's signature on the Affordable Care Act had dried, the Republicans vowed to repeal the bill. Their weapon was "the personal responsibility requirement," otherwise known as "the individual insurance mandate."

Why is it that individual responsibility, a core principle of conservatism, is suddenly so unacceptable for Republicans?

Those who were opposed to the individual mandate took Obamacare to court. They say the individual mandate is unconstitutional.

Is it?

*****

If men were angels, no government would be necessary.

–James Madison The Federalist Papers, No. 51 (1788)

STOP SIGN AND THE INDIVIDUAL MANDATE

Sandy fell backward and broke her neck. She was roller-skating. After the fall, she immediately realized that something was seriously wrong. She couldn't move her arms. She told the people who were trying to help her to call an ambulance. They asked Sandy if she was sure about that because she didn't have medical insurance, and it was going to cost her a lot of money. She told them she had no choice. She was taken to a nearby hospital. An x-ray of the neck spine showed that there was a fracture of one of the vertebrae, and the MRI showed injury to her spinal cord. That explained why she couldn't move her arms. She was flown by helicopter to one of the bigger Level 1 trauma center hospitals, where I was on a neurosurgical emergency call that day.

When I saw her in the neurosurgical ICU, her neck was immobilized in a hard collar. She had what is called Central Cord Syndrome, a form of spinal cord injury that causes weakness, predominantly in the hands. The next day, I did surgery on her neck spine and used a plate and screws to immobilize the fractured vertebra. Over the next few months, she regained all her strength and eventually started to ride her motorcycle again. I did warn her to wear her helmet. She told me, with a smile, that she always wore one while riding.

Sandy owned a small business but didn't have medical insurance; it was too expensive. Since Obamacare was trying to give tax breaks to small-business owners, I asked her what she thought of Obamacare. She said she didn't know much about it, but she didn't like it. I was somewhat surprised. Why wouldn't Sandy like Obamacare when it was trying to help, precisely, people like her? I wasn't sure if she understood the benefits that the Healthcare Act was going to provide for small-business owners. But then, she was not alone when it came to not liking Obamacare without even knowing any details or understanding the benefits. The interesting thing is that they are not displeased with Obamacare; they hate Obama. I was not sure if they hated Obamacare because they hated Obama, or hated Obama because of Obamacare, or maybe both!

I happened to see videos and pictures of rallies protesting Obamacare. People came in droves! They didn't want the government to expand access to healthcare for all Americans. They wanted Obamacare repealed. They said it was unconstitutional and encroached on their freedom. They weren't going to tolerate it. They didn't hide their displeasure for Obama himself, either. Their feelings were clearly displayed on the signs they were holding during the rally. Some of those signs showed more than displeasure for the president; they represented hatred toward him. One sign said, "Obama's plan - White slavery." Another said, "The American taxpayers are the Jews for Obama's ovens," and, of course, there was a sign with Obama in a Nazi uniform with Hitler's mustache that read, "Barack Hussein Obama - The new face of Hitler." Since Obamacare was perceived to be a government takeover of healthcare, there were many signs equating Obamacare to "socialism." One of them read, "Barack Obama supports ABORTION, SODOMY, SOCIALISM, and the NEW WORLD ORDER." There were some more offensive signs than those that are unsuitable to be mentioned here. Then, there were the gun lovers. Their signs included "Guns tomorrow." Some of them came with guns hanging from their shoulders. These were the Tea Party activists. They said that they were taxed enough already. They wanted their Republican leaders to repeal Obamacare.

In fact, not too long after the Obamacare law was signed, twenty-six state attorneys general, mostly Republican, two ordinary citizens, and the National Federation of Independent Businesses joined in filing lawsuits in Florida, claiming that Obamacare was unconstitutional. The plaintiffs objected to two provisions: First, the individual mandate—citizens without insurance are required to purchase it—and second, an expansion of Medicaid—states are required to expand the coverage they offer the poor. On January 31, 2012, Judge Vinson of the U.S. District Court for the Northern District of Florida sided with the plaintiffs and ruled the entire act unconstitutional. The case went to the Supreme Court, which, on June 28, 2012, by a 5-4 decision, upheld Obamacare as constitutional. Chief Justice John Roberts, the conservative, wrote that the individual mandate could be considered a tax and that Congress has the power to mandate a tax. The court did find that the expansion of Medicaid, enforced with a penalty of withholding federal funds, was unconstitutional. Still, the core of Obamacare survived.

As I was following the individual-mandate drama, the hatred of the Republicans and Tea Party activists for Obama and Obamacare didn't make any sense to me. I kept thinking of the stop sign. There are no signal lights at a crossroads where there is a stop sign. The whole idea of a stop sign is that the crossroads are not busy enough to have a traffic light but busy enough to require stopping. Drivers are supposed to make sure that nobody else is crossing the road before crossing it. If they don't do that, then they may get into an accident and kill somebody else, or themselves, or both. It is the responsible and prudent thing to stop, but there are people who won't stop, even knowing that not stopping is bad for them and harmful to others. This is why stop signs remind me of medical insurance. Doctors, hospitals, and eventually all citizens will bear the cost of the medical needs of the uninsured. According to one report, it costs $1,000 per year for each person who pays for healthcare to take care of those who don't.

If citizens were responsible for themselves, there would be no need for the government to impose penalties. Since many are not responsible, the government is forced to act. That's why there is a fine if you run through a stop sign. It is for the benefit of everybody, just like everybody purchasing healthcare insurance.

What is even more perplexing to me is that most of the people who want to repeal Obamacare are conservatives and believe in individual responsibility. There was a man who made just that point while he was the governor of Massachusetts. In fact, he said a system that takes care of people who go to the ER in spite of not paying for healthcare is equivalent to socialism. That's why, in his signature law that provided healthcare to every citizen of Massachusetts, he made sure the individual mandate was a key component.

His name is Mitt Romney. He created Romneycare, the model for Obamacare.

The irony of this is that a conservative idea—the individual mandate—which was championed by many Republicans in the past, embraced by Romney, and later by Democrats in crafting Obamacare, became the very core of the argument to repeal Obamacare. I am astonished that Romney wants to disown his own healthcare plan, which he once considered to be his proudest bipartisan accomplishment. I was a little perplexed by the incongruity: most Republicans not only didn't object to the individual mandate in Romneycare but also nominated Romney to be their presidential candidate in 2012. It seems like they didn't use the same set of criteria when criticizing Obamacare since it is almost identical to Romneycare.

Did Romneycare do so badly after it was implemented that Romney is running away as fast as possible from his own signature and proud accomplishment as governor of Massachusetts?

*****

It is the law that was the source code for Obamacare. It is the law that dare not speak its name. It also happens to be the best thing Mitt Romney will ever do in his life. Without it, I'm not sure how my family and I would live. Why would a man be ashamed of helping so many people?

–Charles P. Pierce "Life Under Romneycare" Esquire, Oct. 2012

ROMNEYCARE

On April 12, 2006, with the stroke of a pen, then Massachusetts Governor Mitt Romney became the first man in the history of America to attempt to bring affordable, quality healthcare to all the citizens of a state. The signing was witnessed by one of the most liberal senators in America, Ted Kennedy, as well as a man from the Heritage Foundation, which is at the conservative extreme of the political philosophical spectrum. Now, that is an example of two political achievements in one shot. It is no ordinary feat, bringing together a liberal idea of universal healthcare and a conservative idea of individual responsibility accomplished through an individual health insurance mandate. Understandably, it was Mitt Romney's greatest achievement, which he was very proud of and of which he really should be.

According to the *Esquire* article by Charles P. Pearce, a citizen of Massachusetts, "The law has succeeded so well that six years into its implementation, 97 percent of the working-age adults in Massachusetts are covered by one form of health insurance or another, as are 99.8 percent of the children in the state. Before the law was passed, 67 percent of the businesses in the state offered health insurance to their employees. That number is up to 77 percent now. The program consistently polls at about 63 percent in its public approval. It has made thousands of lives easier, including my own."

In March 2012, the National Bureau of Economic Research published a study of the impact of Romneycare on the healthcare of people in Massachusetts. The report was very positive: the physical and mental health of the citizens improved. In addition to improvements, surprisingly, there were positive trends in decreasing body mass index and an increase in moderate physical activity. Women, minorities, near-elderly adults, and low-income families had the greatest gains. It seems the law achieved what it was intended to do.

Another important aspect of Romneycare is how it is able to achieve what it does. It uses subsidies and health insurance mandates, both of which the Republicans disapprove of in Obamacare. This disapproval is a philosophical incongruity between the Republican platform and the political history of the man they chose to be their presidential candidate. It is ironic to see Romney bashing Obamacare, knowing that Obamacare is philosophically and operationally identical to his own Romneycare. That is the mother of all political flip-flops. It is a shame that Romney has to resort to bashing what amounts to be his own program, especially knowing that he has helped save many lives and improve the health and well-being of even more lives. I personally have encountered a citizen of Massachusetts who, like me, feels Romneycare is a good thing.

Remember Whitney Gaines, the cancer patient who was asking for help on the streets of Cambridge in front of the Harvard University campus? She told me that Medicare and MassHealth had helped her get the necessary treatment for her cancer. Without those, she would have had no help at all. She told me that the governor of Massachusetts, whose name she didn't know, had made it compulsory for every citizen of the state to have health insurance. She added that it was like having a license to drive; if you're living in the state, then you must have medical coverage. I guess she was talking about Romney and his "individual mandate." She said if you are poor, you go to the state and apply for a subsidy, and you get it. I asked if mandating everybody to have health insurance was a good thing. She didn't hesitate. She said emphatically that it was. She also told me, "Massachusetts is the only state in the country that provides healthcare to every citizen of the state." In fact, her sister brought their mother, who lived in Virginia and got sick, to Massachusetts because she didn't have insurance and couldn't get any medical help in Virginia. Even though Whitney didn't know the name of the man who had improved their lives immensely by making much-needed medical help available, she was grateful to him.

I'm sure Mitt Romney knows that Romneycare is his singular political achievement. Deep in his heart, he must be proud of it and of the good it is doing for ordinary citizens. Why, then, is he disclaiming it so totally? Could it be that he wanted to be the Republican president of the country at any cost, literally, and had to disown ideas of his own that were not popular with the conservatives and embrace their policies? Oh! What the love of political power will do to a man! It can transform him into somebody completely the opposite of who he is at his core, just as Dr. Jekyll could turn into Mr. Hyde. The problem for us with Mitt Romney is that we don't know which of them is going to show up if he is given the ultimate responsibility of presidential power. As Abraham Lincoln said, "Nearly all men can stand adversity, but if you want to test a man's character, give him power."

I think I have an idea which Romney is going to show up. He gave us a glimpse of that Romney in his vice-presidential running mate, Paul Ryan.

Paul Ryan, the architect of the Republican budget plan, wants to revamp and transform Medicare as we know it.

Oh, no!

Currently, seniors love and depend on Medicare. I wonder what the transformed Medicare is going to look like. Will the seniors really be helped or hurt by Ryancare?

*****

The greatest threat to Medicare is Obamacare, and we are going to stop it.

–Paul Ryan vice-presidential-nomination acceptance speech Republican National Convention Tampa, Florida, August 29, 2012

RYANCARE

"Keep government off my Medicare: You damn socialists!" The person holding the sign was most likely a government-hating, Republican, Tea Party activist. I saw this sign at a Tea Party rally protesting Obamacare, urging Republican lawmakers to repeal it. He wasn't alone. Many men and women, young and old, were holding similar signs.

The irony is that these sign carriers were giving a ringing endorsement to Medicare, a federally taxpayer-funded and government-run national health insurance program that helps Americans over sixty-five and those who are disabled. From the signs, it really looked like these activists didn't realize Medicare is a government-run program. If government-hating Tea Party activists like Medicare so much that they don't want any disruption to that "government" system, it must be a really good system.

I'm not surprised that many of those people like Medicare, even though they think anything related to the government is socialism. Medicare is very popular among seniors for a good reason. It's all about providing good service to eligible recipients. It has no interest in making a profit. It doesn't prevent seniors from enrolling in Medicare, even if they have pre-existing conditions.

If Medicare had "pre-existing condition" rules like for-profit health insurance companies, most seniors would be refused enrollment. Instead, 100% of all seniors in America are covered by Medicare. Also, Medicare doesn't drop enrollees from the plan if they get sick. If it did, there would be no seniors in the program because as we age, we are bound to get sick.

However, there is one man who champions the cause of revamping Medicare: Congressman Paul Ryan.

Paul Ryan was not well known to the public before he was nominated as the vice-presidential running mate of Mitt Romney. Within political circles, however, he was known for the Republican budget plan he proposed as a member of the House Budget Committee. He called it *The Path to Prosperity: A Blueprint for American Renewal.*

I'm not sure if he was thinking of prosperity for all Americans. Nonpartisan analysts of this budget say it contains two main underlying principles: (1) stimulating the economy by cutting business taxes, including those of wealthy corporations, and (2) cutting spending. The main way he wants to cut spending is by reducing Social Security and Medicare.

Ryan wants to change Medicare as we know it. Instead of allowing it to remain a not-for-profit government service, he wants to privatize it. He proposes turning it into a system where the government would provide "premium assistance" to seniors—essentially a voucher system. Seniors would then use these vouchers to purchase insurance from private companies. Those older than fifty-five would still have access to traditional Medicare, but those younger would choose between the voucher system and traditional Medicare when they become eligible.

One of the reasons Mr. Ryan wants to privatize Medicare is because he claims it is inefficient. In fact, Medicare is far more efficient than many, if not all, private insurance companies. The administrative costs of major insurance companies range from 15% to 30%, whereas Medicare's administrative costs range between 3% and 5%. This is because most private insurance companies, being profit-oriented, must advertise and market their insurance products. Additionally, they pay lavish salaries and bonuses to their executives, who often travel in private jets. Private insurance companies will never bring their costs down because they prioritize big profits. They are not in the business of healthcare delivery out of compassion or altruism; they are in it to make money.

Medicare has already experimented with a version of privatization. It gave private insurance companies an opportunity to reduce Medicare costs through a program called Medicare Advantage. However, the insurance companies failed to achieve this. It's not hard to see why. Even if they could increase efficiency and reduce fraud more effectively than the current government-run Medicare, they wouldn't return the savings to the government. Instead, that money would go to CEOs as bonuses. The bottom line is that privatization wouldn't save any money for Medicare participants, but it would certainly generate profits for insurance company executives.

The Obama administration recognized this issue. As a result, the funds previously allocated to Medicare Advantage will be redirected to help cover the costs of implementing Obamacare.

Most importantly, Mr. Paul Ryan does not seem to understand that private, highly commercialized, for-profit, greed-driven enterprises are a significant cause of the escalating costs of Medicare and healthcare in America. I'm sure Mr. Ryan believes in the free market and assumes that a competitive capitalist economy can cure the illness plaguing American healthcare. Unfortunately, greedy capitalism is actually the deep-rooted infection—or cancer-causing the illness. I hope he reconsiders and takes the time to understand how the healthcare industry in America truly functions.

Another reason Ryan claims he wants to reform Medicare is to give patients more freedom and choice with their healthcare. Maybe he doesn't realize that, with Medicare, patients already have more choice and freedom than they would with many private health insurance companies. Trust me—I know. I'm a doctor. I get far more hassles from private insurance companies when I try to order the diagnostics or interventions my patients need—HMOs are the worst—than I ever get from Medicare. So, this rhetoric about privatizing Medicare to gain freedom and choice simply isn't true.

Do those government-hating but Medicare-loving Republican and Tea Party activists understand the inflation risk of privatizing Medicare? The amount of premium assistance (voucher) Congressman Ryan is proposing would be fixed, even as the costs of diagnostics, treatments, and pharmaceuticals continue to rise. This means seniors would receive fewer and fewer benefits over time for their fixed premium assistance (voucher). Under such circumstances, I can guarantee that private insurance companies will cut coverage and benefits or shift those costs to seniors through copayments and high deductibles.

If I were a senior, I'd be wary of Ryancare.

Ryancare will never surpass the current Medicare system in providing necessary benefits to seniors.

If this is the case, why do Congressman Ryan and many other Republicans want to transform the highly satisfactory, government-run Medicare into privatized Medicare? Could it be those special interests—pharmaceutical companies, insurance companies, and hospital associations—stand to gain even more than they already do?

Are you kidding me? Of course, they will.

Revamping Medicare is not the only goal of the Ryan Plan, and seniors are not the only group of Americans who will be affected. The Ryan-Romney Plan will also impact millions of Americans relying on Medicaid, the healthcare program for people of all ages who are poor and require financial assistance. The plan proposes cutting Medicaid by approximately $810 billion.

Millions of poor children and adults—the most vulnerable members of society—will lose the assistance they desperately need. Sixty-two million children currently depend on Medicaid. Poor seniors who rely on both Medicare and Medicaid to cover their nursing home expenses will be hit the hardest.

The Ryan budget, endorsed by Romney and many Republicans, seeks to reform Medicaid by introducing block grants to states. Block grants allocate funds for general areas of social welfare rather than specific programs. The result? Medicaid funding, which provides essential help for the poor, will be drastically reduced.

This will happen at a time when more Americans—due to the recession—have fallen into poverty. Since 2010, the number of

Medicaid-eligible citizens has increased by ten million, costing Medicaid an additional $410 million in the fiscal year 2010 alone. This wasn't due to uncontrollable costs; it was because more Americans needed assistance.

Finally, another reason Ryan cites for his draconian cost-cutting measures is the lack of money in the budget. He points to the trillion-dollar deficit and the national debt, which has surpassed $15 trillion—almost as large as the GDP.

Why is there such a massive budget deficit and escalating national debt?

Is cutting Medicare, Medicaid, and Social Security the only way to solve the fiscal crisis we face?

To answer that question, all we need to do is follow the money in the budget to see where it's going.

*****

Some people in Washington want to cut Social Security and veterans' benefits by cutting the cost-of-living adjustment. But there's a better way to cut government debt than cutting Social Security and veterans' benefits: cut the bloated Pentagon budget.

–Robert Robert Naiman Huffington Post, Aug. 30, 2012

BUDGET WARS

The blast occurred right under the middle of the Humvee, punching a hole in the floor and filling the inside with smoke

and fire. Sergeant William Kleindeler, the driver, saw a white ball of smoke rise up in front of his eyes. He was dazed and didn't quite know what had happened, but a voice inside his head told him to get out of the vehicle. He knew he needed to do that, but he couldn't. The voice kept telling him to get out of the vehicle. He tried to open the door, but it wouldn't open. The blast killed three of the soldiers in the vehicle instantaneously. The smoke and fire were getting worse. After a few more tries, the door finally opened. Bill fell to the road and immediately realized that another vehicle might run him over. He rolled to the side of the road into a ditch. He looked up at the Humvee and saw somebody get out of the vehicle, completely engulfed in flames with his arms flailing. Bill shouted at him, "Get down! Get down!" But the body fell on the ground, succumbed to the flames, and died.

All 10,000 rounds of ammunition in the Humvee caught fire and exploded, melting the vehicle. Bill started to feel an excruciating pain in his face. His nose, ears, mouth, and cheeks were all burnt except for his scalp and eyes, which, fortunately, the helmet and goggles protected. Paramedics arrived at the scene, gave him morphine to ease some of his pain, and he was flown to Baghdad and from there to San Antonio, Texas.

Bill was born and grew up in a small Midwest farming town, then he joined the US Army and was deployed to Iraq. He was driving back to base after a medical mission when his Humvee hit the Improvised Explosive Device (IED).

After nine surgeries over eight months, including many skin grafts, Bill was able to head back to his home in rural Massachusetts, where he is now rebuilding his home and his life. All his medical needs, including multiple surgeries and follow-up medical treatments, were taken care of by the government-run Department of Veterans Affairs. He was also able to get some financial assistance to buy a house.

More than 33,000 young soldiers have been disabled in combat in Iraq in the last ten years, and more than four-thousand have died. Around 150,000 Iraqis have died in the war, and more than one-and-half million were displaced from their homes and turned into refugees. The pain and suffering of the Iraqis and the American soldiers is incalculable. We can never estimate its price. But we do know how much the unnecessary Iraq war has cost us monetarily: more than $1.5 trillion and counting. It is a war funded by credit cards, thanks to all the congressmen and congresswomen in Washington, DC, who voted for it, including Paul Ryan. By the way, Mr. Ryan, that's enough money to sustain almost five years of Medicare. Instead, that money has been spent on an unnecessary and horrible war.

That enormous amount of money for the Iraq war motivated me to look at our budget carefully. How are we spending the public's money, especially when we are strapped for cash? Our politicians, who are the government, say the government has not been frugal or responsible. They say that there is no money in the bank, that we are broke, that we are at the edge of a fiscal cliff, just about to fall over the precipice. As I looked at our budget, the first big-ticket item that caught my eye was defense spending. It is the most expensive of all, more than Social Security, Medicare, and Medicaid, although it is less than all of them combined.

However, what I found to be especially interesting is how these expenditures are categorized in the budget. Social Security, Medicare, and Medicaid - the so-called entitlements - are in the "mandatory" expense category, and defense is classified under "discretionary" expenses. There is a reason why they are classified this way, and the categories underscore the fundamental philosophical differences in the nature of these expenditures. Our immediate, individual well-being may not depend on what we are spending for the military, but the social- safety-net spending is essential for the well-being of our citizens, especially in an economy that is in recession.

When we are forced to pinch our pennies, it makes sense to cut the discretionary spending first before cutting the mandatory spending. That has been a time-tested principle of managing one's finances. That is what a wise homemaker will do when faced with economic distress. Unfortunately, politicians have a way of ignoring that age-old wisdom.

Another principle related to tax policy that is being advocated by some politicians also makes me question their wisdom. It is "trickle-down economics," that is, cutting taxes to the wealthy,

who really don't need it, with the hope that the economy will grow and prosperity will trickle down to the hard-working middle class or the poor. This experiment was tested in George. W Bush's presidency. The result was clear: No prosperity trickled down to middle-class or poor Americans. Instead, there was a recession, and many hard-working middle-class citizens became poor and the poor poorer, while the overall wealth of a small percentage of rich people increased. Those politicians who want to continue or enhance such tax policies either don't seem to be paying attention to recent history or have really short-term memory. I also wonder about their common sense.

I asked myself what a loving and wise mother would do when forced to divide up a limited supply of food for her kids. Would she reduce the portions to the already starving and hungry and give generously to the well-fed and satiated? Or would she be fair and do the right thing? She would surely make her priorities reasonable, which, I am sorry to say, does not seem to be the case in the People's House, the House of Congress. Politicians want to give more tax cuts to those who don't need them and reduce the social safety net for those who need it at a time when they need it the most. There is a fundamental philosophical difference between the two parties about how to fix the fiscal crisis we are in. The Democrats say the Republicans are balancing the budget on the backs of the middle class. The Republicans say that Democrats are waging class warfare. I am skeptical that they will be able to find a mutually agreeable solution. It's not just that they don't seem to be capable of working together; they appear to be at war, a budget war.

It seems to me that the only rational, reasonable, and humane policy to pursue is to do less war-mongering and more social healing. I am sure there will be enough money if we spend it right. As a physician, I often remind my patients that "prevention is better than cure." Surely, preventing war and its human and monetary costs is better than trying to cure the physical and psychological devastation and monetary destruction caused by one. Sadly, the truth is that the devastation and destruction that a war causes are actually impossible to "cure."

Any reasonable person is outraged when the so-called fiscally conservative and responsible politicians say there is no money for the social safety net but generously spend on an unnecessary war anyway. They beat the patriotic war drums with unmatched enthusiasm to invade and decimate another country, but I don't see the same enthusiasm on the part of the politicians or corporations when it comes to avoiding the economic destruction caused by irresponsible laws or policies in the financial industry. Do they care about the industrious and productive American citizens pushed into economic hardship as a result of these misguided policies? Some of our veterans whose lives have been changed forever by war are trying to do the best they can to lead as normal a life as possible. They have personally seen the death and destruction of war. They are against war, especially an unnecessary war.

I met an Iraqi war veteran in Washington, DC., who is in a similar situation to Sergeant William Kleindeler in his need for post-war medical treatment and care and who expressed similar concerns.

Geoff was deployed to Iraq, where he sustained a brain injury that made him disabled. When he came back, he thought about what had gotten us into the war and decided that invading Iraq was an unnecessary knee-jerk response to the 9-11 attack. He joined IVAW, Iraq Veterans Against War. When I met him, he was proudly wearing an IVAW T-shirt. He lamented what might have been: What if on 9-12, instead of going to war, we had examined the causes of the attack and responded in a different way, a more humane way? Perhaps we should have launched assistance and help for the needy rather than invasion and destruction. He thought that the world would be better off without the never-ending war that we are currently in. He also noted that he wouldn't be the wounded war veteran he now is. This is a clear example of wasted money on unnecessary war that could have been spent on the social safety net of Social Security and Medicare as well as other important and necessary expenditures like education and national infrastructure. Spending money on the destruction of other nations, which are made up of hard-working, desperate people just like us, rather than repairing our crumbling roads and bridges, makes no sense to Joe.

One thing that he said related to the healthcare he received as a veteran especially caught my attention. He said that being a wounded war veteran, he was glad that he had the government-run VA and Veterans Administration to help him out when he needed it. He was very pleased with all the care that he had received. He was especially thankful that he didn't have to go broke because of his ill health, which was caused by his combat in Iraq. He said that he was very satisfied and happy about the "socialized medicine" that the VA provided him. He felt he wouldn't have been treated as well by the private health-insurance systems that are all about nothing but profit. He hated that private insurance companies tried to ration the care that doctors wanted to provide to their patients. He was well aware of how many times the insurance companies had refused benefits and surgeries, knowing that the patients would die.

He knows the VA is better than a private insurance company because he compares his medical care with that of his sister, who is also a chronic pain patient but who has private insurance. He said there is no comparison between the two systems. His sister does not get the medical care she needs from her private medical insurance. He was angry at all those who say government-run healthcare is bad. He said they didn't know what they were talking about. He knew it to be otherwise out of his personal experience. He is proud to endorse a system similar to the VA for all Americans, a single-payer "socialized" system. He is quite angry with the current system.

He is not the only one who is mad at the current healthcare system and thinks a single-payer government-run system is a better alternative to the present one in this country. There are many doctors who believe the same. They are single-payer advocates, and they are angry. They are really mad.

They are the "mad as hell doctors."

They are getting together and organizing. They want to do something about dysfunctional healthcare in America. They want to help the patients who are sick and suffering but do not have access to decent basic healthcare.

*****

I am mad as hell because, after 25 years of practice, I am convinced that a publicly funded, privately delivered single-payer system is the only alternative. Thank you!

–A "mad as hell doctor" in Portland, Oregon

THE CURE

It was an unusually cold October morning in Washington, D.C. Just the day before, it had briefly snowed, surprising many. No wonder Dr. Margaret Flowers was bundled up in a sweater, a wool cap, and a scarf wrapped tightly around her neck. She needed all the warmth she could get because she wasn't in the cozy confines of her home. Instead, she was living in a tent erected in Freedom Plaza, just a stone's throw from the U.S. Capitol.

She told me she had been living in that tent for weeks. I was impressed but not surprised, knowing her unwavering commitment to the cause of single-payer health insurance for all Americans.

Her dedication was precisely why I was there that morning. I wanted to interview her for my healthcare documentary, which focused on her unrelenting advocacy and activism to bring universal healthcare to all Americans.

I first learned about her from a segment on PBS's *Bill Moyers Journal.* She recounted an incident in which she was arrested while trying to get President Obama's attention. She had gone to the hotel where he was speaking, hoping to hand him information about a compelling idea to reform healthcare in America.

After all, just a few days earlier, during his State of the Union address, the president had said he would be willing to listen to anyone with good ideas about fixing the critical condition of healthcare in the country. Taking him at his word, she prepared a statement about the benefits of a single-payer system and went to the White House to deliver it.

She was denied access, which wasn't surprising. First of all, she wasn't a wealthy, powerful lobbyist. Secondly, the president didn't seem particularly interested in hearing about a single-payer approach. He likely knew there was no political will in the Capitol—and perhaps not on his part either—to pursue such a system in America.

Her failure at the White House motivated her attempt to deliver her message at the hotel. However, being private property, the hotel staff wanted her to leave the premises. She pleaded with hotel security, explaining that she only wanted to hand the president a suggestion. But the hotel called the police, and she was arrested.

When I came across the video of her arrest on YouTube, I wanted to learn more about her. I discovered that she was a pediatrician practicing near Baltimore and trained at Johns Hopkins University. Her elite education clearly demonstrated her intelligence, but her concern for her patients revealed her deep compassion.

She was frustrated by the limitations imposed on her ability to treat patients by private insurance companies. She deplored the questionable morals of these companies, which prioritize profits over patients. She felt they were implicitly forcing doctors to conform to the unethical principles of the for-profit insurance industry, compromising their ability to provide necessary care.

Dr. Flowers realized that the only way doctors could offer conscientious care to their patients was by eliminating the myriad of highly commercialized, profit-driven health insurance enterprises that control thousands of doctors. The only plausible alternative, in her view, is a publicly funded, truly not-for-profit single-payer system, like Medicare—but for all Americans, not just eligible seniors and the disabled.

Dr. Flowers truly and deeply believes that our current profit-driven healthcare insurance system needs to be replaced by a single-payer system like Medicare for all.

Many Americans, however, question whether there is an alternative to a single-payer system. They worry that, unlike the current system, a single-payer system might lack choice and flexibility. Others ask why the existing system can't simply be reformed—made more efficient and less wasteful—rather than replaced.

The billion-dollar question is: Will such a reform be realistically possible?

Consider the report from the Institute of Medicine, which highlighted that healthcare delivery in America wastes $760 billion a year. The report suggests several ways to reduce this waste, but each recommendation has significant challenges.

For instance, the institute recommends streamlining administrative costs to save $181 billion annually. However, as long as private enterprises dominate, administrative costs will continue to include profits and bonuses.

The report also discusses improving hospital efficiency to save $80 billion per year. While hospitals are already working on this, the savings often go toward bonuses for CEOs rather than reducing overall costs.

Another suggestion is to decrease the costs of episodes of care, but with everything overpriced by greedy manufacturers, it's unclear how costs can realistically be lowered.

The institute urges preventing avoidable admissions or readmissions, which currently cost $68 billion annually. However, hospitals often make more money with more admissions, and many doctors find it easier to send patients to the ER or admit them to avoid malpractice lawsuits. As a result, these admissions are likely to continue.

The report proposes reforming medical liability, but that's a tall order when Congress is dominated by representatives who are lawyers.

Finally, the report calls for improving the targeting of costly services. But what does that even mean in practice?

Preventing medical errors, which cost $12 billion annually, is another recommendation from the Institute of Medicine. Absolutely!

Preventing medical errors is crucial—not just to save money, but more importantly, to save patients' lives. However, when the current system permits a high patient-to-nurse ratio for economic reasons, and hospital administrators push doctors to see as many patients per hour as possible—essentially treating their offices like assembly lines—the likelihood of serious fatigue increases, keeping the medical error rate alarmingly high.

Additionally, continuity of care is at risk, leading to further medical errors. This happens when shift-work hospitalist doctors, employed by hospital administrators, clock out at the end of their shifts and transfer patient care to the next shift's doctors.

The institute also advises preventing fraud and abuse, which currently cost $10 billion annually. But, greed-driven individuals will always find ways to defraud the system. For instance, consider the Columbia-HCA hospital conglomerate, once run by Rick Scott, which was fined $1.7 billion for Medicare fraud.

Finally, the report suggests increasing shared decision-making to save $9 billion annually. Yet in a system where administrators make decisions without consulting doctors—or ignore doctors' input entirely, relying instead on "yes-men" doctors on decision-making committees—it is unrealistic to expect improved shared decision-making.

The Institute's recommendations are nearly impossible to implement within a fragmented, profit-driven healthcare system that thrives on the status quo and is fueled by greed. No wonder Dr. Flowers firmly believes that the only true solution is a single-payer system, which would eliminate the greed embedded in our current commercial medical enterprises.

As the president delivered his speech inside the hotel, Dr. Flowers waited outside with a large banner reading, *"Letting You Know: Medicare for All,"* hoping the president might see it as his motorcade passed by.

What began as voluntary, part-time, state-level advocacy for a single-payer system had become a full-time occupation for her. She left her medical practice and fully immersed herself in her mission to bring single-payer healthcare to America.

When I met her, she was in Washington, D.C., to give a talk at a workshop during the annual conference of Physicians for a National Health Program (PNHP) in October 2011.

PNHP is a Chicago-based organization with more than 14,000 members, including doctors, nurses, and non-medical citizens who believe a single-payer system is the cure for the problems plaguing healthcare delivery in America. I was eager to attend the PNHP conference.

One speaker from Canada discussed the decent healthcare system in his country. A radiologist from England spoke about her fight against the conservative government's attempts to privatize healthcare in England, which would undermine the highly popular NHS (National Health Service). She believed such privatization would destroy the universally admired healthcare delivery system in her country. She noted that the British are so satisfied with their healthcare system that it is even more popular than the royal family. Adding a touch of humor, she joked that saying such things might land her in the Tower of London as punishment.

Dr. Arnold Reiman was also at the conference, and I was especially keen to talk with him. I read his book, *Second Opinion*, which detailed the history and evolution of healthcare delivery in America and how profit-oriented commercial enterprises took over the service of healing. He had personally witnessed these changes and documented them in his book.

Dr. Reiman argued that the failure of physician leadership in America, along with their opposition to any government-run single-payer system, created a void. This void was filled by greedy businessmen—and some businesswomen—who built the Medical-Industrial Complex, profiting from people's ill health.

I asked him if there was a feasible solution to this crisis. He said that while a solution is possible, it would be difficult to achieve.

Dr. Reiman explained that dismantling the for-profit Medical-Industrial Complex is essential. This would require gradually phasing out, through legal means, the for-profit private insurance companies, hospitals, diagnostic centers, medical laboratories, pharmaceutical companies, and nursing homes.

Most importantly, doctors would need to support the elimination of the fee-for-service system. This system incentivizes unnecessary, ineffective, and duplicated diagnostics, prescriptions, and procedures. In a fee-for-service system, "more care" pays doctors more, increasing the utilization of medical resources—even if it doesn't lead to better care or improved outcomes. He firmly believed that a not-for-profit, government-run, single-payer system was the solution.

Hearing this, I felt a moment of pessimism. We live in a capitalist country where many are skeptical of government involvement in individuals' lives. It's a country where many people are highly individualistic, believing in self-reliance and self-sufficiency, and where the competitive free market is seen by many as the cure for all ills—even in medicine.

However, that conference was not a place for pessimism about the possibility of achieving single-payer healthcare in America. Many of the doctors who gathered there believed it was possible.

All that needs to be done, they said, is to expand Medicare. It is already a payroll-tax-funded, single-health-insurance plan that covers 100% of citizens over the age of sixty-five, but it could easily be expanded to include everyone. Medicare operates very efficiently and is much cheaper than any private insurance plan because it eliminates the element of profit. Additionally, it has significant leverage to negotiate lower prices from pharmaceutical companies.

Many capitalists might argue that expanded Medicare would be unfair because it would create a monopoly. However, many insurance companies and hospital associations already operate in monopolistic ways. Doctors have no real bargaining power against insurance companies that continually cut payments to physicians while raising premiums for patients.

Meanwhile, larger hospitals acquire smaller ones, fail to make their costs and pricing transparent, and continue to increase profits. The uninsured, much like consumers in markets dominated by monopolies, are left with no choice but to pay whatever they are charged.

Some people express excessive concern about the government's susceptibility to fraud. However, fraud can be addressed and controlled. Even if additional funds were allocated specifically to combat fraud, Medicare would still be far cheaper than commercial insurance companies.

"Medicare for All," the PNHP doctors argued, is highly feasible and could be relatively easily accomplished. Many countries already have such a system: Sweden, England, Finland, and our neighbor, Canada. As in these countries, there could be coverage for "catastrophic" and predetermined healthcare needs for everyone.

However, many Americans believe a single-payer system would limit choices and alternatives. These individuals prefer options and often point to countries like France and Australia, which operate a two-tier system. In this model, basic universal healthcare is funded by taxes and provided by the government, while anything beyond that requires individuals to purchase additional private insurance or pay out of pocket.

Then, there are countries like Germany and the Netherlands, which mandate the purchase of insurance. In these nations, insurance companies are heavily regulated to prevent excessive profits. Other medical industry enterprises are similarly regulated to avoid price gouging.

I was still pessimistic that any of these systems could be implemented in America. After all, our healthcare delivery is deeply commercialized. But then I met two women doctors—one an M.D. and the other a Ph.D. in Social Anthropology. One of them wore a button on her sweater that read, "I Love Single Payer."

Both were from Vermont. One of them told me that Vermont would soon become the first state in America to implement a single-payer system.

What? A state with a single-payer system in capitalistic America? I never thought that would be possible in a country where healthcare delivery is so profit-driven. Yet Vermont is already on its way to providing universal healthcare to all its residents through a state-run, publicly funded, single-payer system.

I knew I had to talk to them and learn more about how they achieved this milestone.

*****

We gather here today to launch the first single-payer healthcare system in America, to do in Vermont what has taken too long – have a healthcare system that is the best in the world that treats healthcare as a right and not a privilege.

–Gov. Peter Shurnlin Montpelier, Vermont May 30, 2011

THE LITTLE ENGINE THAT COULD

One sunny morning in Vermont, the Green Mountain State, a few hundred people gathered on the front steps of the state house. It was going to be a historic day. These citizens were about to witness an accomplishment by Vermonters that would be the first of its kind in any state of the United States of America. That's a big accomplishment for a small state. Vermont is the smallest landlocked state in the country. Its capital, Montpelier, is the smallest of all the state capitals. Burlington, the largest city in Vermont, is the smallest of the largest cities in any state in America.

The governor was about to sign into law Green Mountain Care, the first single-payer healthcare law in America. Vermont would become the pioneer in providing healthcare to all the citizens of a state through a publicly funded system. Dr. Alice Silverman, one of the two women from Vermont that I met at the PNHP conference in Washington, D.C., told me it was "about time for that to happen."

Dr. Silverman is a psychiatrist, and she has treated many citizens of Vermont, mostly hard-working farmers with significant anxiety. They were very anxious about how they would cope financially if they faced a serious medical illness. Their inability to afford medical insurance was more worrisome to them than their fear of the disease itself. They were concerned that a single illness during the later stage of their lives could destroy their life savings. They might lose everything paying for medical expenses, making them financially unstable at a time in life when they needed and were expecting some rest, relaxation, and peace of mind.

They were being realistic in fearing that medical expenses might make them go bankrupt. In America, the number-one cause of personal bankruptcies is medical costs. Dr. Silverman felt sorry for the psychological suffering of her patients. She began to think about possible healthcare solutions for all the uninsured or inadequately insured Vermonters. She heard about PNHP seventeen years ago and learned more about single-payer health insurance. She became convinced that it was the solution, providing a just system that could bring accountability to healthcare delivery. She joined and is still an active member of PNHP. She was proud to be in Vermont as the state began a new chapter in the healthcare history of America.

But how was Vermont, a small state, able to achieve such a monumental feat?

Dr. Deborah Richter and Dr. Ellen Oxfeld, whom I met at the PNHP conference, were the two leading activists who laid the groundwork for it to happen.

Dr. Richter originally practiced medicine in Buffalo, New York. Many of her patients were young people suffering and dying from the consequences of not having preventive and early healthcare. Some had juvenile diabetes (JD), a preventable and manageable disease if medical intervention is early. One young man who was her patient with JD became blind and died at the age of twenty-five. A young female patient, also in her twenties, died after delivering a premature baby, surely preventable if she had had adequate prenatal care.

Dr. Richter became interested in a single-payer health solution but found it difficult to achieve in a large state like New York. She moved to Vermont, feeling that the smallness of the state might offer a logistical advantage. In Vermont, while still practicing, she gave hundreds of presentations to educate the public, as well as politicians, about the justness and benefits of a single-payer system. Then, she met Dr. Oxfeld, who teamed up with her in the single-payer cause. They became the two single-payer missionaries.

I was fortunate enough to meet Dr. Oxfeld personally at the PNHP conference in Washington, D.C. She is a professor of anthropology at Middlebury College in Vermont. Her travels around the world gave her the opportunity to see how many less-prosperous countries are able to provide better and universal healthcare. This realization made her become a tireless activist for the cause of bringing affordable healthcare to all Vermonters. She believes single-payer is the answer. Together with Dr. Richter, as part of the group "Vermonters For Healthcare For All," she informed and organized the state's citizens to activate, agitate, and protest in order to bring about a single-payer system for her state.

A law, Act 48, for publicly funded single-payer health insurance, was introduced in 2010 in the legislature of Vermont. Dr. Oxfeld's group kept a close watch on the progress of the act. Any time the legislation encountered roadblocks, the group informed and educated its members to respond appropriately to address the roadblock, whether the problem was a particular politician or otherwise. The members organized protests and also more formal communications with their congressional representatives. Their enormous hard work paid off. The act was passed into law by a vote of 94-49. A Democratic House, Senate, and governor of Vermont made it possible. She told me the law is a road map to bring single-payer to Vermont by 2017. The supporters want to have it happen sooner, but a waiver from the federal government would be needed to do so. Even if they have to wait until 2017, Vermont would still be the first state in the country to enact a single-payer system—an enormous achievement in America.

Small the state may be, the achievement of ensuring every citizen has health insurance provided by a single-payer is an enormous accomplishment. It reminds me of the story of the little engine that could. In fact, Vermont has a history of being the first to do big things in the nation. After joining the Union, it was the first state to abolish slavery. Wow! The little state is actually a big and great pioneer in America when it comes to doing the right thing!

Dr. Richter has some reservations about the law but will take the victory for now. She feels that Green Mountain Care is not truly a single-payer system because private insurance companies are still allowed to operate in Vermont. That may be the reason those commercial insurance companies have not gone "all out" to oppose Green Mountain Care. They did not launch a campaign to defeat the Democrats instrumental in passing the law.

The Vermont accomplishment is an encouragement to single-payer activists and should make them optimistic, but the million-dollar question is: Will it be inspirational enough to make single-payer happen at a national level? If America, like many other developed nations, can bring about affordable, universal, quality healthcare, then that will be a huge accomplishment. Many Americans and their elected lawmakers equate government involvement in healthcare to socialism or communism. A single-payer system in America would represent a philosophical shift for a society dedicated to free-market capitalism, which, by the way, I believe is not truly free.

I do want to mention that many people in America may not be aware that there is legislation, H.R. 676, introduced in the U.S. Congress for national single-payer health insurance.

The introduction of that legislation is a start, but the journey to reach the ultimate passage of the law will be hard, fraught with opposition from rich and powerful special interests profiting from the current system. Dr. Richter feels, "There is no shortcut to a national single-payer healthcare system, and politicians with the best of intentions will not gently enact it. There is no way to avoid a head-on collision with the parasitic, for-profit insurance industry to put them out of business once and for all. Let's stay on that road."

She knows that difficult road well. She has traveled down that path to achieve the precursor of single-payer in Vermont. Not that she is satisfied with it. "In my opinion," she says, "it's better to have a fight for national legislation like H.R. 676, as proposed by Rep. John Conyers, that really does create a single-payer system and abolishes the private insurance industry than to have a fight over a piece of state legislation with no funding mechanisms, is riddled with numerous bureaucratic roadblocks, and makes vague promises to enact what the majority of people want—healthcare as a human right for all."

As Governor Shumlin signed the Green Mountain Care Act into law, all the proud Vermonters who gathered for the occasion on the steps of the Vermont State House posed for a group picture. They held a large banner that read, "Health care is a human right."

America is at a philosophical crossroads on the issue of providing quality, affordable healthcare. One of the roads continues in the direction of greedy capitalism that we have been traveling along, which has benefited a few and failed many. The other road leads to a just and fair single-payer system that provides decent healthcare, and thus peace of mind, to all its citizens. The free-enterprise commercialized system has been tested and proven to be ineffective, creating a country where health is a privilege for those who have plenty of money.

This creates two Americas as far as healthcare is concerned, with poor people receiving inadequate care. Everybody knows this is unfair, but many Americans consider a single-payer government system to be socialist and communist, and they abhor it. So, alternatives and variations have been advocated. Many Americans who are concerned about the current healthcare system but believe in having some choice favor the idea of a two-tier system, where all Americans are guaranteed basic healthcare, but those who have money can afford more choices and expedited medical care, as in France and Australia. This is like the difference between first-class and economy-class services when flying. Both classes get the same final outcome—reaching the destination—but the first class gets advantages, comforts, and extra perks. The economy class gets peanuts, literally, while the first class gets Pinot Grigio and Champagne. This kind of two-tier system is still unfair.

Many other schemes have been offered, especially with the goal of controlling costs due to excessive utilization by doctors or by patients of employer-provided health benefits: HMOs, PPOs, Managed Care, Health Savings Accounts, Capitation, Co-payments, and outright restriction and denial of benefits by insurance companies. None of these schemes has led to universal healthcare at a reasonable cost. The only other choice is the one based on the principle that healthcare is a basic human right and all Americans should be treated equally: a government-sponsored single-payer system. Any objective analysis of the problem of healthcare in America would yield the same necessary solution. We are at the crossroads of greed and fairness. Which road are we going to take as we look to the future of healthcare in America?

For many Americans who are highly individualistic and skeptical of the role of government, the choice of a federal single-payer system that provides affordable, universal healthcare is like a bitter pill. Even so, a balance between individual freedom, individual responsibility, and the role of government is not unreasonable. If we want to rescue America's dying healthcare system, we may have no choice but to swallow that bitter pill.

Healthcare in America is in critical condition. Will Americans accept the bitter pill of choosing the right path? And even if they accept, will it be possible to rescue American healthcare from the clutches of a political system beholden to profit-driven and greedy special interests?

*****

The mind is everything. What you think, you become.

–Buddha.

LIFE, LIBERTY, AND THE PURSUIT OF HAPPINESS

October 6, 2011

Washington, D.C., USA

It was a beautiful fall afternoon—sunny, not too warm, not too cool. I was happy as I walked out of my hotel to go for a stroll on K Street, a stone's throw from Lafayette Park, which is just across from the White House. Only a few minutes earlier, the annual conference of the American Association of Neurological Surgeons had ended. Every neurosurgeon is required to attend sixty hours of "Continuing Medical Education" per year to maintain board certification in neurosurgery. I was glad that the conference was over because I had enough education over the past few days. I wanted to have some fun.

Washington, D.C., is a beautiful city. Each time I've gone there, I've enjoyed it very much. When I visit the National Mall, I experience the magnificence of America, the greatest democracy on the planet. It is awe-inspiring to see, at one end of the mall, the Capitol, where lawmakers wield immense power, along with the president in the White House, not too far away. In the middle of the mall is the Washington Monument, commemorating a man who fought for and led the independence struggle against the unjust British rulers.

At the other end is my favorite memorial, the Lincoln Memorial. I don't think I've ever missed paying a visit to the imposing statue of Lincoln whenever I visit D.C. I've always been an admirer of Lincoln, a man who truly represented America's core conviction—the belief that all men and women are equal. He proclaimed emancipation for slaves in the spirit of that conviction and paid dearly with the ultimate price: his life. I love his famous words about democracy: "government of the people, by the people, and for the people."

Ironically, that day, as I was walking on K Street, I came across people gathering in McPherson Square to protest America's growing economic inequality and injustice. Their common cause, which brought them together, was the complaint that America, the greatest democracy, hasn't fulfilled its democratic principles. They felt that, instead of being the government for all the people, it has been for the benefit of a few—the 1% that is rich and powerful. These protesters were in the square to start a movement.

"Occupy D.C."

That's what the red letters on the huge white banner said. The protesters were shouting, "We are the 99%" and "This is what democracy looks like." There were signs that said, "The hungry. The poor. The 99%" and a banner that asked, "Who owns your senator?" The Occupy Movement was spreading throughout America. A few months earlier, it had started on Wall Street to protest the widening gap between the rich, the top 1% of Americans, who are getting richer, and the rest who don't benefit to the same extent. Many Americans felt they weren't benefiting at all and, instead, were losing economic ground after the bursting of the housing bubble and the subsequent recession.

Many middle-class Americans have lost their jobs, health insurance, and then their homes. They woke up one day to discover that they were poor. Many CEOs of banks, big corporations, pharmaceuticals, health insurance companies, and large hospitals seem to have been immune to the economic collapse. They made a lot of money and laughed all the way to the bank. The middle class, who suffered the brunt of the recession that the banks had caused, were upset and wanted the government to know that the current capitalist democracy was not working for them. They wanted their voices heard, some of which I had a chance to hear personally.

That's where I met many occupiers who were dissatisfied with the state of the union. Joe, the man who was depressed and almost committed suicide, was one of them. He wanted to let the country know that very expensive healthcare prevents access to affordable, quality healthcare for many Americans. He was especially angry at the greedy and highly profitable pharmaceutical companies that benefit from the high prices of life-saving drugs, knowing that many can't afford them. He wanted the politicians to do what is good for the public, not what is good for their re-election. He even made a sign on what looked like a piece of cardboard that said exactly that.

Simon was another young man who wanted to say a few things about his plight as far as access to decent healthcare is concerned. He has epilepsy and is uninsured. He wondered why a wealthy country that has some of the best technology and innovation in medicine fails to provide universal healthcare to all its citizens. He constantly worried about not having health insurance. He knew that he could end up on the street anytime, helpless and hopeless, if he developed any other medical problem that he couldn't afford treatment for.

Caren, a young protester who had just graduated from college, said that healthcare in America is great for people who are rich but not for those who don't have money. She was happy, though, that she was able to stay on her parents' insurance, thanks to Obamacare. She gave a grateful "shout-out" to Obama.

The Occupy DC rally is also where I met the Iraq war veteran who was against war. He was grateful for the government-run Veterans Affairs medical care, which has been taking care of his post-traumatic stress and the other injuries he suffered in combat. Being a man of peace, I appreciated the words on his T-shirt: "Iraq Veterans Against War," when one of the men there told me a huge peace march was about to start at Freedom Plaza, a few blocks away.

I had to attend that. I almost ran to Freedom Plaza.

I saw a lot of people there—young and old, disabled and in wheelchairs, as well as healthy—who were shouting slogans, waving signs, and some carrying banners. Many had lost jobs. Students were protesting the weight of their student loan debt. Gan Golan from Los Angeles had a ball and chain in one hand and a sign in the other that read, "Master of degrees: Shackled by debt." Different people had different grievances, their signs reflecting their concerns: "Health care for all," "Health is a human right," "People over profits," "Justice for all," "Human need, not corporate greed," "Stop wars," "Out of Afghanistan, now!"

There were Veterans for Peace and moms and aunts holding signs telling the government not to deploy their sons and nephews. They said, "Enough!" I was delighted to come across a girl walking with my favorite sign: "Make love, not war." As a neurosurgeon who has worked to save lives from injury, one life at a time, and knows how hard it is to do that, I've always hated war. It kills or disables countless numbers of soldiers as well as civilians, so many can die with just the press of a button. I had to stop her and ask if I could take a picture of the sign. She obliged, and I felt happy.

Looking at that gathering, with all those concerned citizens taking time and making an effort to shape the political process, I felt inspired. Here was democracy at work! Here was freedom of speech!

Then, a huge, special American flag caught my eye, a flag with the stars replaced by peace symbols. I loved the beautiful way that flag expressed my own love of peace. I had to talk to the lady who was carrying it. Her name was Carol Gay.

Carol is from Brick, New Jersey. She is the president of the New Jersey Industrial Union Council and also chair of New Jersey Labor Against War. She is truly a woman who loves peace. She told me that she had been working to end the war for ten years. She thought that all the money we spend on destructive war could be spent wisely and better for humane purposes, like healthcare for all, education, roads, schools, and jobs, rather than killing. She was upset that the rich were getting richer and the poor were getting poorer. She wanted people to understand that the rich could be taxed to pay their fair share for the benefit of the entire nation and that there is money in the country for everybody to have a decent quality of life if only the politicians and the public would have the will to realize it. She said that Medicare, for example, is very efficient in providing healthcare to all seniors, and its administrative costs are only 3%. Compare that to the 30% of private insurance companies, which includes huge profits and bonuses for their CEOs. For that reason, she has been fighting to realize "Medicare for all."

As I was talking with her, I heard what sounded like war drums, gradually getting louder and louder. I looked in the direction of the sound and saw drummers beating a huge drum on wheels and leading a march of protesters toward the stage in Freedom Plaza. They were carrying a huge banner that looked like the paper on which the Constitution was written. The script on that banner, created to resemble the one in the Constitution, began with big words that said, "We the corporations ..." As the marchers reached the stage, I saw a similar huge banner in the back of the stage that started with the words, "We the people ..." Those two banners clearly reflected what was happening in the country—the conflict between the rich and powerful corporations and the people who are experiencing hopeless economic despair. The marchers were enthusiastic and energetic and were dancing until Dr. Margaret Flowers came on the stage with a megaphone and said that they were all gathered there to "stop the machine," an all-encompassing machine that includes many aspects of society, like the war machine that proliferates and benefits the war industry with unnecessary wars and now with drone attacks. A huge model of a drone was on a pole next to the stage, with some clothes on the ground dipped in red paint, symbolic of the blood that is being spilled as a consequence of war and drone attacks. She also talked about stopping a corporate machine, which makes a few people richer at the expense of many people's jobs, healthcare, and quality of life.

She talked about stopping the corrupt political machine that creates laws for rich and powerful special interests while marginalizing the middle class. Some of the corporate leaders and politicians who operate this machine blame the ordinary citizens for their own difficult financial situation, but Dr. Flowers thought it was the system that had failed the people. In her opinion, the political machine and some of the mainstream media may claim and want the people to believe that "the poor Americans" are responsible for their own economic dire straits, but it is the greedy corporations that have outsourced jobs, put their profits and wealth offshore, almost bankrupted the financial system by creating a toxic housing bubble, and then got bailed out by taxpayers when that bubble burst. They then paid huge bonuses to themselves with the bailout money. For what—ruining the country?

What Dr. Flowers and Carol Gay had said resonated with my own observation and understanding of how healthcare is an integral part of the socio-economic and political system of the country and why many feel helpless to face the powerful machine of corporations and corrupt politicians.

As a doctor concerned with the lack of access for millions of Americans to affordable, quality healthcare, I am convinced that the entire medical-industrial complex needs to be revamped if we want to provide access to quality healthcare to all citizens. This will probably require a political and economic system overhaul. There are many players in the medical industry who say they wish for the system to be changed but continue with the current ways for profit. But mere wishing will not bring about change. As Gandhi said, "We must become the change we want to see in others." The greedy for-profit pharmaceuticals, insurance companies, hospitals, lawyers, device manufacturers, medical business enterprises, as well as doctors, are not going to change themselves. The system, which is so profitable to them, has to be changed by others.

Who is capable of doing that?

The two main players that have that ability are the concerned doctors and the citizens. Together, they can bring about the necessary change. The citizens have the voting power to replace a corrupt political system that is perpetuating this highly commercialized, for-profit medical industry. Doctors will have to help the citizens understand the special-interest ills of healthcare in America as well as provide leadership to bring about the change. For too long, doctors have yielded the leadership role, to their own detriment, to the predatory special interests of the medical-industrial complex. It is time for doctors to stop being short-sighted, too self-centered, and egotistical and unite if they truly want to wrest control from those special interests for their own good as well as for the benefit of their patients who trust them with their lives. That will happen when the majority of doctors wake up and remember that they have sworn the Hippocratic oath, that they became doctors in the first place to help and heal the sick, not to profit from them. As Dr. Flowers said, "We (the doctors) have a responsibility for our patients, and there is a lot of healing that needs to be done in this country."

I hope the enthusiasm and energy of the activist citizens continue to inspire the rest to participate in the democratic political process to change the existing political system. As Dr. Reiman said, "The politicians need one thing to get re-elected. They need votes." The public holds in their hands the power to change the country and, thus, their own lives. John Locke, whose philosophy inspired the founding fathers to include "life and liberty" in the Declaration of Independence, said, "It is the duty of the citizens to vote the politicians out of power when they fail to deliver their responsibilities."

As I was about to leave Freedom Plaza, I saw a mother dancing with her young son, who had a smile on his face. At that moment, I realized how important it is to have a peaceful and healthy America for this and all the coming generations.

We can achieve universal healthcare in this country. It is already done in many other civilized and industrialized countries that are less wealthy than America. Now is an opportune time to act because our economic crisis brings the problems that have been killing healthcare slowly and insidiously out into the open. It has never been more urgent or possible than now to achieve affordable, universal healthcare for the well-being of all Americans.

The sad story of Kelly Parker exemplifies the need to fix the system, and it cannot be ignored anymore. There are many similar stories, but her story tugged at my heart when I heard about it. Kelly is a single mother of two who bought her small dream home on the west side of Detroit. Because her mortgage doubled, she was not able to pay her taxes, and the county put her house up for auction. She was not going to let that happen to the house for which she had worked so hard. In order to discourage any potential buyers, she painted graffiti all over the outside walls of the house: "Our house," "We are not leaving," and "Mine."

As if the threat of losing her home was not enough to deal with, she learned a few days prior to receiving her eviction notice that she had brain and lung cancer. She could not afford to pay all the expenses to take care of her medical problem on top of the money needed to keep her home. Her friends were trying as best as they could to help her out.

Her story makes me think about why a social safety net is essential for every citizen. When hardship hits, we may not have the means to withstand it, and our family and friends may not be able to help us sufficiently. We should then be able to count on the compassion of all the citizens that, collectively, will have created a nation with a safety net that supports us through the hard times.

I can't imagine the sadness and suffering Kelly Parker must have gone through. In spite of everything, she was determined to fight to keep her house while fighting to save her life. Even though she knew her children might lose their mother to cancer eventually, she didn't want them to lose their homes, too. She wanted that house to be passed on to them as her gift, in addition to the gift of life that they received from her as their mother.

Kelly Parker's struggle for her health, economic stability, and peace of mind is the story of many Americans. Unless we, as a nation, choose the path of compassionate care that treats all Americans as equal, we are headed for the inevitable deterioration of our great nation. The country is burdened by escalating healthcare costs, and that burden is only getting heavier. We have to do the right thing for the sake of our health and well-being and that of our children. We must strive to achieve a true democracy for all the people, as envisioned by Abraham Lincoln.

I wish for peace and love and, of course, health for all. Only with good health will there be a possibility for us to have personal freedom as well as the liberty of a healthy society to pursue a meaningful and fulfilling life of happiness, for health is the greatest wealth.

-The End-

www.ingramcontent.com/pod-product-compliance
Lightning Source LLC
LaVergne TN
LVHW050916210926
848482LV00012B/464